Schriftenreihe Neurologie
Neurology Series 18

Erlo Esslen

The Acute Facial Palsies

Investigations on the Localization and Pathogenesis of Meato-Labyrinthine Facial Palsies

With a Foreword by U. Fisch, Zurich

With 127 Figures

Springer-Verlag
Berlin Heidelberg New York 1977

Privatdozent Erlo Esslen, M.D.
Division of Neurology, Kantonsspital Aarau, Switzerland

The investigations were performed at the University Hospital of Neurology, Zurich, Switzerland.

ISBN-13: 978-3-642-66536-3 e-ISBN-13: 978-3-642-66534-9
DOI: 10.1007/978-3-642-66534-9

Library of Congress Cataloging in Publication Data. Esslen, Erlo. The acute facial palsies. (Schriftenreihe Neurologie). Bibliography: p. Includes index. 1. Paralysis, Facial-Etiology. 2. Facial nerve-Diseases-Diagnosis. 3. Facial nerve-Surgery. 4. Electrodiagnosis. I. Title. II. Series. [DNLM: 1. Facial paralysis-Etiology. 2. Facial nerve-Pathology. 3. Constriction, Pathologic-Complications. 4. Herpes zoster-Complications. 5. Labyrinth. 6. Petrous bone. WISC344 Bd. 18/WL330 E78a]. RC418.E87. 616.8'7. 67-55687.

Offset printing and bookbinding: Brühlsche Universitätsdruckerei, Lahn-Gießen 2123/3130-543210

Foreword

I have been privileged to work with Dr. Esslen for more than ten years and to have witnessed how surgical progress combined with accurate clinical and electrophysiological investigations have revolutionized the diagnostic and therapeutic approach to the paralysed face.

The long journey of the VIIth nerve through the temporal bone has been considered for years responsible for the particular liability of this nerve to acute palsies. The disappointing results obtained with surgical decompression confined of necessity to the mastoid and tympanic segments of the fallopian canal led us in the sixties to apply modern otoneurosurgical techniques in order to achieve total exposure of the intratemporal course of the facial nerve. At that time Esslen started to record with surface electrodes the compound action potential evoked by maximal percutaneous stimulation in representative areas of the facial muscles. With this method, called electroneuronography, exact determination ot the percentage of degenerated nerve fibers could be achieved in the early stages of the palsy. Precise electroneuronographic criteria for the selection of patients requiring surgery in order possibly to improve the outcome of their disfiguring paralysis were worked out. At surgery direct stimulation of the totally exposed intratemporal portion of the facial nerve was used for the first time in combination with electroneurography in order to determine objectively the degree of the lesion. In contrast to what has been believed for years the pathology related with acute facial palsy has been found to be situated in the majority of the cases at the entrance and not toward the exit of the fallopian canal. Although further studies are necessary to establish without question the value of timely surgery, the present monograph establishes without doubt that, in order to be effective, it has to be performed in the most hidden labyrinthine and meatal portions of the facial nerve. In any case, the electroneuronographic criteria indicate that less than 5% of the patients can be considered as candidates for surgery. In view of the localisation of pathology familiarity with the most modern otoneurosurgical procedure is an essential prerequisite for a successful operation.

The work of Esslen has deeply extended our knowledge on the natural history of the most common acute facial palsies and has established valid criteria for surgical indications. There is no doubt that Esslen's monograph will remain for years to come the basis for a logical therapeutic approach to the acutely paralysed face.

Zurich, March 1977 U. Fisch

Preface

This treatise is the result of 10 years of close cooperation between neurologist and otologist. The cooperation began with the question of how the results of "decompression" of facial nerve could be assessed. This intervention had then for more than 10 years been part of the repertoire of otologic operations. It implies the opening of the tympanic or mastoidal section of the fallopian canal and slitting of the epineurium. The indication for this intervention was, however, rather vague and opinions on the most appropriate time varied considerably among otologic surgeons.

We tried to answer the question of the usefulness of decompression of facial nerve by combined clinical and electromyographic investigations. Several years of work on this revealed that decompression of the facial nerve did not improve the prognosis. This was confirmed some time later by other investigators (Naumann et al., 1968; Adour and Swanson, 1971).

This disappointing result was enhanced by the fact that the exploration of the facial nerve after opening of its canal did not show any impressive alteration of nerve tissue suggesting that one had found the site of the essential pathogenetic processes causing palsy. For both of these reasons, the ineffectiveness of decompression as well as the vanishing evidence of the underlying pathogenetic concept, this intervention was given up in 1967 in Zurich.

The new technique of transtemporal opening of the internal auditory channel and of the fallopian canal, introduced in Zurich in 1968, completely changed the situation. The first probatory openings of the internal auditory channel in cases of herpes zoster oticus, later of Bell's palsy as well, revealed an enormous edema and hemorrhage, infarction of the facial nerve just before the entrance to the fallopian canal, and a severe strangulation of the nerve at the transition of the relatively wide fundus of the internal meatus acusticus and the much narrower canal of the facial nerve. The grossly bulging facial nerve could not enter its proper canal without a two to threefold reduction of its diameter. These observations induced new concepts about the localization and the essential pathogenetic factors involved in different types of acute facial palsies. Considering the severe morphologic alteration of the facial nerve at the entrance to its canal it was assumed that this was also the site of functional disturbance. In order to test this assumption, the facial nerve was electrically stimulated along its whole course through the petrosal bone after opening of the internal auditory channel and the fallopian canal and the evoked compound muscle action potential of facial muscles was recorded.

The results of these investigations and the *integration* of morphologic and electrophysiologic findings form part of the first section of the monograph.

In relation to the new operative technique and the outlook of a very much improved method of decompression of the facial nerve, an ever growing need for more reliable methods of pre- and postoperative evaluation and documentation of the *functional* and morphologic state of the facial nerve became obvious. All electrodiagnostic methods hitherto applied did not allow the establishment of a profile of the day-to-day alterations of the facial nerve and did not make possible a close follow-up of the natural history of facial palsies of different genesis. The application of an electroneurographic method adapted especially for this purpose has led to the discovery of "rules" of this natural history. The knowledge of these rules has created a new basis for earlier and more reliable prognoses in acute facial palsies. Furthermore it has established an essential similarity of natural history in facial palsies of different etiology.

I am indebted to Prof. Baumgartner, Head of the University Hospital of Neurology, Zurich, for kind support of this work.

Zurich, March 1977 E. Esslen

Contents

1. Introduction

1.1. Anatomical Considerations

1.1.1. Course of the Facial Nerve in the Petrosal Bone (Fig. 1)

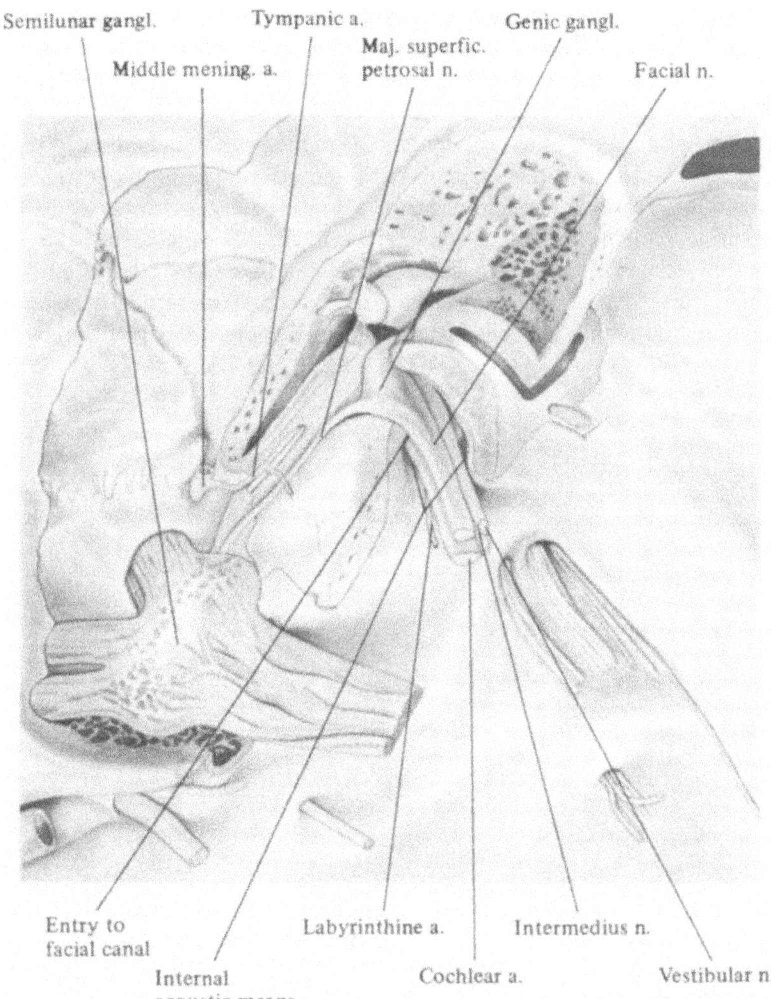

Fig. 1. Middle cerebral fossa. Dissection of internal acoustic meatus after removal of its roof

On opening the roof of the internal acoustic meatus, routinely done in transtemporal decompression (see 2.1.0), the first structure to be seen is the facial nerve. A little behind this nerve and deeper one half of the vestibular nerve can be recognized, while the other half of the nerve, covered by the facial nerve, cannot be seen. Between the two nerves lies the intermedius nerve (or pars intermedia), not visible from above. The cochlear nerve is totally covered by the facial nerve and can be inspected only partially by gently removing the facial nerve. Approximately 12–19% of the lumen of the internal auditory channel is occupied by the facial nerve.

All three nerves have a meningeal "glove finger" enclosing them. At the fundus of the acoustic meatus, the facial nerve enters its proper bone channel. Even in this channel the nerve may be followed by a meningeal extension. In this way the cerebrospinal fluid can reach the proximity of the geniculate ganglion. At the entry to the facial or fallopian channel the intermedius nerve is completely integrated into the facial nerve, and its fibers can no longer be distinguished from the rest of the facial fibers (Sunderland and Cossar, 1953).

The facial channel has a length of approximately 30 mm. It is generally divided into three segments (Fig. 2): The labyrinthine segment (2,5–6 mm) runs from the entrance of the facial channel to the geniculate ganglion, and the tympanic or horizontal segment (8–11 mm), from the geniculate ganglion to the lateral semicircular canal. There the nerve changes direction from horizontal to vertical and descends to the stylomastoid foramen. This is the third segment (9–12 mm) called the mastoidal or vertical segment. The geniculate ganglion, containing the cells of taste fibers, is approximately 1.8 mm long.

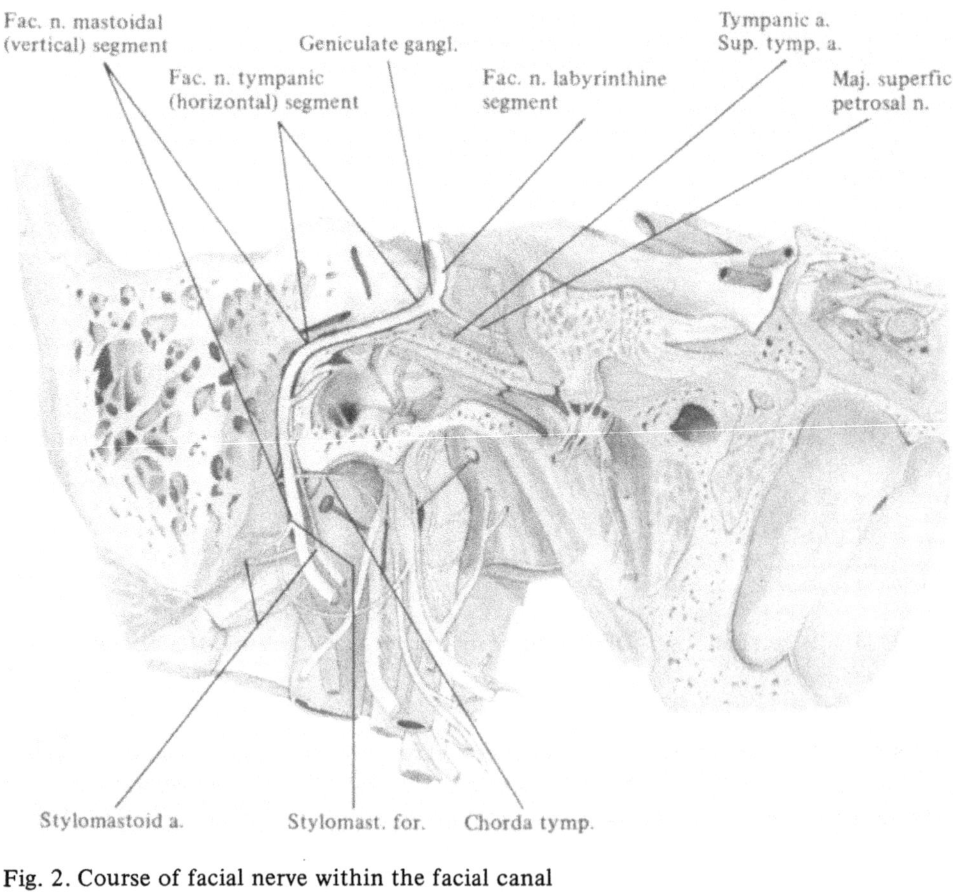

Fig. 2. Course of facial nerve within the facial canal

The ratio of nerve diameter to the one of the bone channel has been repeatedly investigated. The statement of Cawthorne (1946), that there is a narrowing of the facial channel toward the stylomastoid foramen could not be confirmed by later investigators (Lindeman, 1960; Dobozi, 1973). The same holds true for the description of James (1961) of a thickening of the nerve sheath at the stylomastoid foramen, an observation not validated by later investigators. In general, the facial nerve occupies 25–50% of the lumen of the bone channel.

According to the investigations of Dobozi (1973) the narrowest part is not at the *distal* but at the *proximal* end of the fallopian channel. This remarkable communication is based on measurements of 28 petrosal bones (Table 1). It corresponds with the impression one gets by the operative exposure of the facial nerve at the fundus of the internal acoustic channel and labyrinthine segment of the facial channel (Fig. 3).

Table 1. Mean diameter of facial nerve and fallopian channel in millimeters

	Facial nerve	Fallopian canal	Difference
Labyrinthine segment 5–6 mm	0.85±0.07	1.02±0.08	0.17
Tympanic segment 8–11 mm	1.12±0.09	1.53±0.14	0.41
Mastoid segment 9–12 mm	9.94±0.05	1.48±0.12	0.54

By courtesy of Dr. Dobozi.

Even under quite normal conditions there seems to be a certain tapering of the nerve at the transition of the internal auditory channel and the labyrinthine segment.

Vascularization of Facial Nerve

Considerable attention has been paid to the vascularization of the intratemporal segment of the facial nerve in search of a "vascular factor" explaining the genesis of facial palsy in particularities of vascular supply. Reviews on this subject have been given by Zülch (1970), Devriese (1972), and Miehlke (1973). The interest of the authors has been mainly devoted to epineural vessels and anastomoses. The question, however, of intraneural microcirculation and its impact on pathogenesis has obviously been neglected. In Section 1.2.1. therefore this aspect will be discussed further.

The vascular supply in the meatal segment of the facial nerve has been thoroughly investigated by U. Fisch (1968). It is provided by the labyrinthine artery, deriving as single or paired vessels from the inferior anterior cerebellar artery. Thus this section of the facial nerve is supplied via the basilar artery. In the literature it is not uncommon to read of a so-called internal auditory artery, but this vessel is unknown to anatomists. The other two vessels stem from the system of the external carotis. A branch of the medial meningeal artery enters into the facial channel together with the major superficial petrosal nerve and provides principally the tympanic section of the nerve, but also the distal part of the labyrinthine segment. The epineural blood supply of the mastoid

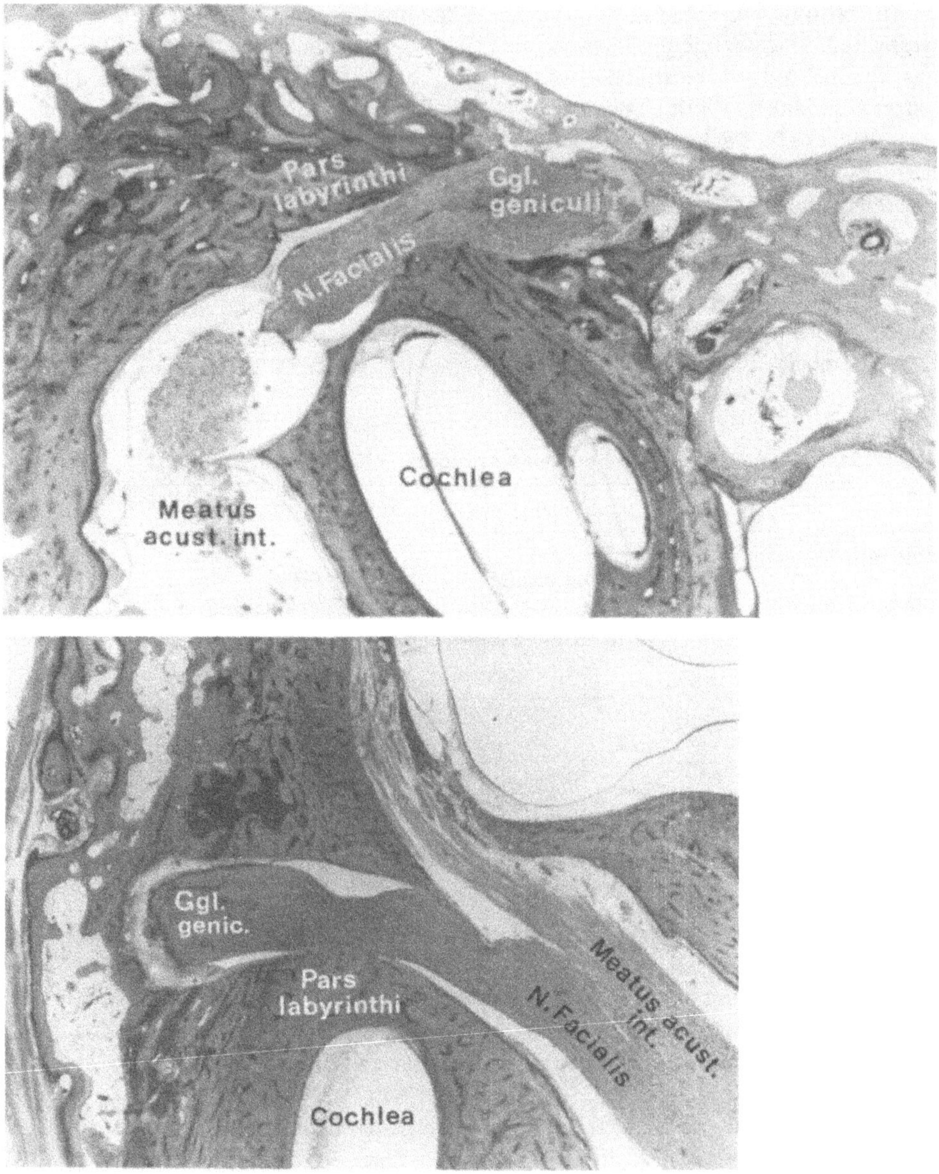

Fig. 3. Dissection of petrosal bone. Entry of facial nerve from internal acoustic meatus into the facial canal (courtesy Dr. Dobozi)

section is provided by the stylomastoid artery. Between the latter and the aforementioned arteries, numerous anastomoses exist. Nager and Nager (1953) have described a number of additional anastomoses. According to the evidence recently presented by Guerrier, there do exist anastomoses with the vascular system of the internal carotid artery, a finding of particular interest.

1.1.2. Composition and Fiber Spectrum of Facial Nerve

The facial nerve contains motor, sensory, and vegetative (secretory) fibers. By comparing the number of cells in the geniculate ganglion and facial nucleus, van Buskirk (1954) has calculated that the motor part of the nerve consists of approximately 7000 fibers. Thus one may assume a similar number of motor units in facial muscles. The 7000 motor fibers represent 58% of the total amount of nerve fibers. The remaining 42% are composed of the preganglionic parasympathetic fibers for salivary and tear secretion (24%) and taste fibers (18%). The diameters of the motor fibers range from 4 to 14 μ with a peak between 7 and 10 μ.

1.1.3. Intraneural Topography of Facial Nerve

Some authors have attempted to find out if a regular somatotopic pattern of nerve fiber bundles corresponding to the different facial muscles and muscle groups exists. Investigations on the nerves of the extremities indicate that the somatotopic principle, so important for the arrangement of structures in the central nervous system, does not play an important role in peripheral nerves (Sunderland, 1968). This holds true especially for the proximal nerve segments leaving the plexus. Further distal, the diffusely mixed nerve fibers are gradually collected to funiculi until they form individual branches, leaving the nerve trunk to innervate the corresponding muscles. The formation of the intraneural plexus has considerable practical importance as it limits the possibilities of interfunicular nerve transplantations when large segments between peripheral and proximal nerve stump have to be bridged. The same considerations are valid for the facial nerve, too, as modern microsurgical technique permits nerve grafts in the fallopian channel as far as the internal acoustic meatus (Fisch, 1973).

Some authors have claimed the existence of a regular intraneural somatotopic arrangement of nerve fascicles for the principal facial muscle groups (perioral, periorbital, frontal region: Miehlke, 1958, 1973; Hoffmann, 1924; Canuyt, 1922). However, there is no agreement among these authors with respect to the configuration of this pattern. According to Miehlke, the nerve fibers for the perioral muscles occupy the lateral (tympanic) sector, those for the frontal muscles the medial nerve sector, and the fibers for the periorbital muscles lie between these two nerve sectors, whereas Hoffmann describes these in the opposing sequence.[1] The most extreme position in this respect is held by Chouard et al. (1969, 1973), who designed an exact intraneural topography of the facial nerve. The fibers to the orbicular eye muscle occupy, according to these authors, the center of the facial nerve. For this arrangement they offer a teleologic interpretation: the fibers for the vitally most important function of facial muscles, lid closure, are the best protected ones.

Sunderland and Cossar (1953) on examination of 13 human facial nerves could not find any regular intraneural topography: "In our material plexus formations in the extracranial portion of the nerve trunk had so mixed the fibers representing individual branches that, at the stylomastoid foramen, each funiculus contained fibers from each main branch given off distal to this point."

1 The view of Miehlke is, however, strongly supported by May.

The same conditions are valid as well for the nerve segment in the fallopian channel, with the difference, however, that in this segment there is no recognizable subdivision in individual bundles of funiculi. Under the microscope, the whole nerve appears to be a single nerve bundle. Sunderland and Cossar state "The greater superficial petrosal branch joined the facial nerve at the geniculate ganglion and there were no special features which permitted the identification of its fibers in the parent nerve proximal to this level. Nor could the fibers comprising the nervus intermedius of Wrisberg be isolated in that portion of the facial nerve contained in the facial canal proximal to the ganglion".

Nevertheless, Sunderland and Cossar admit that the distribution of facial nerve fibers may not be absolutely random, but that there could be a certain aggregation of defined fiber groups in definite nerve sectors. Apart from the above-quoted, rather contradictory arguments for the formation of the intraneural plexus and the mixing of nerve fibers in facial nerve, based on different morphologic methods, there is far more convincing evidence on other lines for lack of intraneural topography. Assuming the topographic principle were valid as strictly as is maintained by Miehlke, Chouard, and others, one would expect that after the separation of the nerve branches distal of the stylomastoid foramen the single nerve branches could contain only fibers of one muscle or at most two neighboring muscles. This, however, is not so. The systematic stimulation of peripheral facial branches performed on more than 50 patients on the occasion of the so-called selective partial section of facial nerve branches (Fisch and Esslen, 1971) has shown that the single peripheral facial nerve branches contain fiber components for very different facial muscles as far as the distal nerve segments. Fiber bundles, innervating perioral muscles for instance, frequently leave nerve branches going to the orbicular eye muscle, only a few centimeters before reaching this muscle, and change over to nerve fiber bundles directed definitely to the mouth. The same holds, vice versa, for fiber bundles supplying the orbicular eye muscle.

The intraneural plexus formation can thus be traced right up to the periphery of the facial nerve. In fact, the plexus formation seems to be more pronounced in this nerve than in the distal segments of arm and leg nerves. This peripheral plexus formation could be observed in each case of the patients operated on one or both sides for hemifacial spasm or of blepharospasm. A striking finding was the great variability of the pattern of the plexus, not only with respect to different individuals but also to both halves of the face in one person.

1.2. Evaluation of Present Views on Etiology and Pathogenesis of Acute Facial Nerve Palsy

Several extensive reviews of the literature referring to this subject have been published (Zülch, 1970; Devriese, 1972; Miehlke, 1973) which may be consulted for general aspects. In the following section several somewhat neglected aspects are to be discussed.

1.2.1. Idiopathic Facial Palsy (Bell's Palsy)

The pathogenetic concept of idiopathic facial palsy formulated by Kettel (1947), Hilger (1949), Sullivan and Smith (1950), and repeated by many others is still considered to be valid though slight additions have been made. It is based on the experimental work of Denny-Brown and Brenner (1944a, b), who concluded that nerve conduction block due to nerve compression was not directly caused by the mechanical effect but by the ischemia provoked by the compression of the nerve vessels. Hilger, Kettel, and others assumed the following sequence of processes occurring on the facial nerve: local spasm of arterioles in the territory of the external carotis, affecting mainly the vertical (mastoidal) segment of facial nerve. This *primary* ischemia triggers off the following processes: transsudation → increase of intraneural pressure → impeding of the venous and lympathic drainage → growing edema of nerve → further increase of intraneural pressure → block of arterial bloodstream → *secondary* ischemia leading to nerve palsy. This sequence of events may be called the principle of *primary* and *secondary* ischemia.

The duration of the secondary ischemia determines the degree of facial palsy and especially how many facial fibers will degenerate. The opinion that mainly the vertical (mastoidal) segment of the facial nerve is affected by these processes was strongly held by Cawthorne et al. (1960). Miehlke, however, has in recent years laid increasingly more emphasis on the horizontal segment too (Miehlke, 1973). One of the main arguments for this view is the observation that the nerve fibers after slitting of the nerve sheath protrude profusely into their intraneural bed. Sunderland, however, pointed out already in 1946 that this can be observed on normal facial nerves, too, which corresponds to the author's own experience.

It is important to realize that this pathogenetic concept and its localizatory correlates were developed at the time when only the vertical (mastoidal) and part of the horizontal segment of the facial nerve were accessible by operation for observation, whereas the more proximal nerve segments remained inaccessible. What was observed in the more distal segments was, as we shall see, nothing but *the remote signs of the decisive pathogenetic processes occuring at the entrance to the facial channel* (see Sections 2.2.0–2.2.3).

Frequent trials have been undertaken to substantiate concepts developed in human pathology by experiments on animals. The efforts were above all directed at developing a model for ischemia, simulating as far as possible the conditions in the human facial nerve. Ischemia was usually produced mechanically by ligating the nerve or by liquid pressure. Other procedures were based on pharmacologic methods, e.g. the local injection of vasoconstrictor substances, or on physical agents such as heat and cold. One of the best developed models of investigation was presented by Devriese (1972). He injected a liquid under supersystolic and superdiastolic pressure into the facial nerve of cats some millimeters proximal to the stylomastoid foramen. The effects of this procedure on the nerve were controlled and observed by stimulation of a peripheral nerve branch and recording of the compound action potential of these fibers on the tympanic segment of the nerve. With this method Devriese was able to produce reversible and irreversible blocks of nerve conduction and, perhaps even more important, he could indicate with considerable accuracy the percentage of conducting to nonconducting fibers by the difference in amplitude of the compound action potential before and after nerve compression. His statement that changes in amplitude of the compound action potential are a far better indicator of changes of impulse conduction of a population of nerve fibers than latency is of particular interest with respect to our own investigations (3.1.0).

Out of the rather voluminous literature on experimental models only those communications have been selected, which elucidate a special aspect. Boyle (1967) produced facial palsies by ultrasonic radiation of the nerve at the horizontal semicircular canal of macacae. This procedure provokes vasodilation and intraneural hemorrhages corresponding to the changes seen in the operative microscope in the fundus of the acoustic meatus in man (see 2.1.2). The author in addition performed mastoidal decompression of the nerve on 12 animals without significant differences in comparison to the spontaneous course.

Another interesting experimental procedure was applied by Coassolo (1952, 1952 a, b) contributing to the much discussed problem of the etiologic significance of exposition to cold as causal factor of the idiopathic facial palsy. He desensitized rabbits against horse serum and exposed the extratemporal segment of facial nerve to strong refrigeration by applying ice. Only desensitized animals developed facial palsy. Intravenous injection of procaine 5 min before the application of cold prevented the nerve palsy.

All these experiments, interesting as they are, cannot answer the question as to how representative they are with respect to pathogenesis of human idiopathic facial palsy. There can be no doubt that the experimental procedures mentioned above cause alterations in nerve vessels and even ischemia. Does this sufficiently substantiate the denomination of idiopathic facial palsy as ischemic facial paresis (Miehlke, 1973)? In facial palsy due to herpes zoster infection, ischemia is also an important and perhaps decisive pathogenetic factor (see 2.1.2, 2.2.2) and the same holds true with great probability for facial palsies on the basis of polyradiculitis und lymphocytic (viral) meningitis. It is not the intention of this monograph to discuss extensively terminologic problems. Undoubtedly, the concept of "idiopathic" facial palsy is also very unsatisfactory, but it is accepted as provisional until the etiology or something more specific about this disease is known. If, according to Hilger and many others, vasospasm is the decisive initial pathogenetic process, it would be far more logical to speak of an angiospastic instead of an ischemic facial palsy. Many etiologic factors are supposed to provoke spasm of arterioles including toxic, allergic, endocrine, and even psychic ones (Miehlke, 1960, 1973).

One should be aware of the many unproven assumptions inherent in these hypotheses. The facial nerve is very well vascularized in its intratemporal course by three regional arteries (see 1.1.1). This is very extensive for a distance of 3–3.5 cm and certainly more than is available for other peripheral nerves. The median and ulnar nerves have no regional vessels in a considerable part of human beings between axilla and elbow (Sunderland, 1944, 1968). The blood supply is in these cases guaranteed exclusively by the intraneural microcirculation (intrinsic system). Besides the intraneural capillary system, forming a kind of plexus, the epineural anastomoses of the facial nerve represent an additional safety factor. This holds at least for the two distal arteries. Only between the proximal and medial regional arteries there may be no vascular anastomoses, according to the investigations of Blunt (1954).

According to the thorough experimental work of Lundborg (1970) the intraneural vascular system (intrinsic system) alone is capable of guaranteeing the blood supply for nerve segments of at least 15 cm in length. With these findings he confirms the results of some earlier investigators. Thus, the intraneural vascular system of the facial nerve should easily be able to compensate the interruption of two or even three regional epineural arteries. This compensation should be all the easier as the interruption of the three regional arteries due to vasoconstriction can last only a few hours. It is nowhere indicated how long it must last until the primary ischemia provokes an edema of the facial nerve and thus initiates secondary ischemia. We must try to find an approximate answer in experiments on animals. Lundborg in his monograph (1970) made a valuable contribution to this question. He produced ischemia by compressing the thighs of rabbits and examined the extra- and intraneural circulation and microcirculation of the compressed and ischemic segment of the ischiadic nerve as well as of the peroneal nerve, exposed only to ischemia. For the evaluation of the alteration of the nerve he measured impulse conduction and permeability of the walls of the vessels applying the Evans blue albumin test. He found differential changes in nerves exposed to the combined effect of pressure and ischemia compared to the nerves suffering only from ischemia. Thus, Lundborg was led to distinguish both states as some earlier authors had already done, whereas in practically all comprehensive reviews on pathology of facial nerve the opinion of Denny-Brown and Brenner (1944) prevails, that damage to nerves caused by compression was in fact the result of the concurrent ischemia (see Miehlke, 1973). A minority of authors, however, had always held the view that compression damages the nerve directly by its mechanical component. This view was recently supported by Ochoa et al. (1973) by a striking discovery: they observed invagination of the myelin sheath at the node of Ranvier at the site of the steepest pressure gradient. This invagination cannot be caused by ischemia but only by the mechanical force itself.

Lundborg's findings, too, give evidence for differential effects of nerve compression and ischemia. His most important points are: The nerve segment exposed only to ischemia regained excitability even after a duration of 6–8 hrs of ischemia, and the compound action potential reached its former amplitude, whereas nerves exposed to the combined effects of compression and ischemia definitively lost excitability after 4 hrs. Disturbances of permeability of the intraneural vessels could already be observed on the compressed and ischemic nerve segments after 4 hrs, whereas they did not occur in the solely ischemic nerve until after 8–10 hrs.

The intraneural micro-circulation has an astonishing capability for recovery even after hours of ischemia. Intravital microscopy has shown formation of some microthrombi after acute ischemia leading to transitory obstruction of vessels. These microthrombi tore loose from the walls of the vessels after some seconds and then were released into the free bloodstream. Only rarely did they happen to fix again to the walls, and they could even pass through narrow vessels due to their plasticity.

Electron microscopy, too, revealed severe alterations in the endothelium of intraneural vessels after ischemia of 10 hrs duration. The epineural vessels, however, were more susceptible, and after ischemia of 4 hrs, the micro- und venous macro-circulation did not completely recover. At the same time considerable extravasates of marked albumin could be observed in the fluorescence microscope. These alterations did not cause an increase in intraneural pressure. This happens only when damage to intraneural vessels surpasses a critical level, beyond which the permeability of the vascular walls increases and intraneural edema appears.

Lundborg's investigations give an idea of what questions a detailed, empirically oriented presentation of pathogenesis of facial palsy should answer.

Returning once again to the hypothesis of the initial vascular spasm as primary pathogenetic event, such a spasm must obviously fulfill the following conditions: It must last several hours. It must be total, that means, the blood supply of all three regional arteries must be so efficiently interrupted, that even a small residual blood volume, necessary to maintain the basic metabolism, could not circulate. Is this a proved fact? Or is it at least highly probable?

Such an extensive vasoconstriction is practically only possible by maximal stimulation of sympathic nerves. The vasoconstriction must be rather strictly limited to the intratemporal course of the facial nerve, as otherwise additional symptoms of vasospasm are to be expected. In experiments on animals (Lundborg, 1970), it has been possible by means of microscopy to observe a conspicuous slowing of the intraneural blood circulation on strong stimulation of sympathetic nerves. But this retardation lasts only 40–50 s, then a "break-through phenomenon" occurs, and part of the vessels dilate despite continuing stimulation, and the bloodstream increases again. The reduction of the bloodstream cannot be called a real ischemia even during the phase of maximal vasoconstriction. Ischemia is characterized not by anoxia alone but also by the interruption of transport of metabolites, by shifts of electrolytes from the intra- to the extracellular space etc., all of which are injurious to the endothelium of vessels. Stimulation of sympathetic nerves only causes hypoxia. The plasma stream as well, though reduced, is never interrupted, so that some transport of metabolites is always guaranteed.

In view of this resistance of intraneural vessels to ischemia, it cannot be easy to damage so seriously the endothelium by the acute sympathicomimetic vasoconstriction that a pathogenetically relevant intraneural edema develops.

1.2.2. Herpes Oticus with Concomitant Facial Palsy (Ramsey Hunt Syndrome)

The viral etiology of herpes oticus is clearly proven. Neither a morphologic nor a serologic difference has been found between the virus of herpes zoster and chicken pox, so that identity of both is generally assumed.

In literature the view is stressed that this disease is in fact an encephalomeningomyelitis, or even more precisely, a dermomucosa-neuro-ganglio-radiculo-myelo-meningoencephalitis. This is correct considering the evidence of the histopathologic findings. The emphasis on the encephalomyelitic component, however, easily leads to the misunderstanding that facial palsy accompanying in 60% of all cases herpes oticus was the symptom of an encephalitis. But all evidence indicates a viral neuritis with intraneural hemorrhages and profuse perivascular infiltrates of lymphocytes and plasma cells (see 2.2.0 and 2.2.2).

The pathogenetic processes decisive for the degeneration of facial nerve are rarely discussed in detail. It should be mentioned, however, that Hunt, who erroneously attributed all herpes oticus cases to an affection of the geniculate ganglion, suggested already in 1907 that the facial nerve would be compressed by the swollen ganglion.

1.2.3. Bilateral Facial Palsies

The bilateral, nonsymptomatic facial palsies do not represent a uniform disease. Most frequently they are manifestations of a lymphocytic meningitis or of polyradiculitis. Practically all lymphocytic meningitis, characterized by a benign course, is of viral etiology. Occasionally, even idiopathic facial palsies may affect first one and then the other side in one patient in such close temporal succession that one may talk of bilateral facial palsy, though this signifies a rather loose application of terms. In bilateral facial palsies due to lymphocytic meningitis or polyradiculitis the palsies of both sides follow each other in a rather short time interval, ranging from some days to not more than 3 weeks. Thus, they fall into one and the same phase or cycle of disease. With an increasing interval and no additional bridging symptoms, suggesting a meningitis or polyradiculitis, one is led to assume, per exclusionem, that it is a question of a succession of idiopathic facial palsies. The prolonged time interval suggests that the succeeding facial palsies are not manifestations of one and the same cycle of disease. One must rather assume that alterations of the interior milieu increase the susceptibility for facial palsies, comparable perhaps to the phase of increased susceptibility to influenza. In case B5 something like that could have happened, whereas case B2 must be considered a borderline case.

The group of bilateral facial palsies of different etiologies has been included in this monograph for two reasons: To look for possible differences in the course of the disease during the acute phase in comparison to idiopathic facial palsies and to trace the variations in evolution between the two affected facial nerves.

2. Investigations, Part I: Intratemporal Stimulation of Facial Nerve for Localization of Conduction Block in Idiopathic Facial Palsy, Herpes Oticus, and Melkersson-Rosenthal Syndrome

2.1. Operative Access to the Internal Auditory Channel and Other Intrapetrosal Sections of Facial Nerve

In the "classical" decompression introduced by Kettel, Jongkees, Miehlke, and others in different countries during the last 25 years, the facial nerve is exposed in its vertical, and eventually also in its horizontal segment, i.e., distally from the geniculate ganglion. The technique of transtemporal access to the middle cranial fossa, however, permits the exposure of the nerve in the internal auditory channel as well as in the proximal (labyrinthine) section of the facial canal as far as the geniculate ganglion and some millimeters beyond. A comprehensive description of this intervention, introduced by House (1961), has been given by U. Fisch (1970, 1973). In the following the main steps of this intervention are recapitulated.

The labyrinthine and meatal segments of the facial nerve are approached through a craniotomy of 3 x 4 cm in the temporal squama, giving access to the middle cranial fossa. The dura is not opened, and the temporal lobe overlying the roof of the internal auditory channel is carefully lifted. After orientation from certain anatomic landmarks the bone overlying the geniculate ganglion is removed. From there the labyrinthine section of the facial channel is opened and finally the roof of the internal auditory channel is removed.

After these preparations, the extension of dura and arachnoidea, enclosing the nerve, can be split. In this procedure some cerebrospinal fluid drains off (see 1.1.1). The final step is the splitting of the nerve sheath. Now the nerve can be inspected from the internal acoustic pore as far as a few millimeters to the geniculate ganglion. If exposure of the more distal segments of the facial nerve is required, this can be subsequently done via the transmastoidal approach.

2.1.1. Intraoperative Stimulation and Recording Technique

Method

The intraoperative stimulation of the facial nerve has been performed by means of very fine tweezers with electrically insulated blades. The tweezers could be correctly placed by visual control through the operative microscope. The nerve was held with slight pressure between the two blades of the tweezers. Flow of current was from one blade to the other, i.e., transversal through the nerve. In this way the greatest intensity of current could be concentrated on the smallest space. Thus a nerve segment of approximately 1 mm length was stimulated, allowing a very precise localization of the site of stimulation. Current loops, falsifying the results, could thus be avoided. For stimulation, square wave impulses of 0.1 ms duration were applied. The required stimulus intensity to reach just maximal stimulation was adjusted by visual control on the screen of the recording instrument. Generally 3–4 volts were sufficient. Then the stimulus intensity was increased 20%, to be sure that all excitable nerve fibers would discharge. Great care was taken never to increase stimulus intensity to more than the indicated values in order to avoid current loops outside the nerve segment just in between the two blades of the tweezers. To be sure of this, a test stimulation of the major superficial petrosal nerve was applied at a distance of 1 mm from the geniculate ganglion. The stimulation of this sensory nerve cannot cause discharges of facial motor fibers as long as there is no spread of current.

The stimulation rate was 1/s. Only compound action potentials showing no variation in amplitude and latency during 10 repetitive stimuli were accepted.

Recording Technique

In the majority of cases coaxial needle electrodes were applied for recording. The electrodes were inserted in the perioral muscles and fixated before operation. In some cases additional recording was done with surface electrodes. For recording a Medelec electromyography unit was employed. The time base was generally set at 2 ms, sometimes at 1 ms. An amplification rate corresponding to 100, 200, and 500 μV/cm was used, depending on the ratio of degenerated to blocked fibers.

Sites of Stimulation

1. 1–2 mm distal to geniculate ganglion.
2. At the geniculate ganglion itself.
3. 1 mm proximal to the geniculate ganglion.
4. Immediately distal to the entrance to the fallopian channel.
5. In the fundus of the acoustic meatus.
6. Midway between the internal acoustic porus and the entrance to the fallopian channel.

In the following tables, for the sake of clarity, the latencies of only 4 sites are indicated:

1. Distal to the geniculate ganglion.
2. Proximal to the geniculate ganglion.
3. Immediately distal to the entrance to the fallopian channel.
4. In the fundus of the acoustic meatus.

The distance between the different sites of stimulation could not be kept constant in the different cases. The distance between the first and second site varied 3 mm, between the 2nd and 3rd site 2 mm, and between the 3rd and 4th site 2–3 mm. These small variations in the distance between stimulation sites are not important for the results.

2.1.2. Results of Intraoperative Stimulation of Facial Nerve in the Internal Acoustic Meatus and Facial Canal. Aspect of the Facial Nerve Under the Operative Microscope

Summarizing the contents of Tables 2.1–3, the most striking result is the correspondence between the morphologic aspect and electrophysiologic measurements, both indicating that the pathogenetically relevant processes take place in the fundus of the acoustic meatus and in the labyrinthine segment of the fallopian channel, i.e., at the transition of the nerve from the relatively wide acoustic meatus to the narrowest segment of its intratemporal course. Surprisingly this holds true for idiopathic facial palsy as well as for herpes oticus. Two cases of Melkersson Rosenthal syndrome show similar findings. The first case of herpes oticus, operated on early (C. D.), showed hemorrhage, swelling, and strangulation in the same manner and intensity as the cases of idiopathic facial palsy. In case 2, where exposure of facial nerve was not done until the 33rd day of palsy, the most severe changes had already disappeared, but the pathologic findings could still be unequivocally localized at the entrance to the facial canal, while at the geniculate ganglion and more distally nothing abnormal could be observed.

Morphologic Aspect

The aspect of the nerve through the operative microscope at 20–25 fold magnification is of striking uniformity in all cases, where exposure is performed during the first 2 weeks after onset of palsy. The following phenomena can be regularly observed:

1. An engorgement of the vessels of the meningeal nerve sheath as well as sanguine imbibition of connective tissue and nerve tissue protruding after splitting of the nerve sheath. This sanguine imbibition of connective and nerve tissues is so marked that it reminds one of hemorrhagic infarction. This is most conspicuous in the fundus of acoustic meatus, but can be followed up into the labyrinthine segment of the nerve. Only some cases show slightly increased injection of vessels to the geniculate ganglion. Proximal to the meatal fundus, the hemorrhagic invasion varies in extent. In some cases it could be observed already at the internal acoustic pore, the maximum, however, was always at the fundus. All cases of idiopathic facial palsy and herpes oticus showed profuse hemorrhages, though in the latter case they were perhaps even more extensive.

2. Each of the 16 cases showed a pronounced swelling of the nerve together with its sheath. Frequently a balloonlike swelling could be observed and the swollen nerve seemed to fill the whole fundus, pushing the vestibular nerve aside. By pulling apart the facial nerve the vestibular nerve could be inspected revealing in some cases a furrow of strangulation. The white coloration of the compressed vestibular nerve contrasted strikingly with the reddish facial nerve. The swelling of the facial nerve prevented in most cases the inspection of the cochlear nerve.

3. The enormously swollen facial nerve suffered regularly a strong strangulation at the entrance to its proper bone canal. After opening of the entrance to the facial canal, the originally white strangulated nerve segment rapidly became red and more voluminous. This process could be so fast, that it was not always possible to evaluate the color of the labyrinthine segment of the nerve before beginning the decompression. The opening of this segment of the canal cannot be abrupt. Instead, the bone roof must be removed section by section. The intraneural pressure of the labyrinthine nerve segment was increased, for after splitting of the nerve sheath the enclosed nerve fibers not only protruded over the sheath, which can be observed in normal nerves as well, but even over the lumen of the bony canal.

Electrophysiologic Findings (Fig. 4)

1. The electrophysiologic investigations on the exposed nerve hint at the proximal part of the labyrinthine segment as the site of the decisive functional disturbance, i.e., the 1–2 mm immediately after the entrance of the nerve in its channel. The biggest change in amplitude took place regularly between the stimulation sites 3 and 2. Thus the conduction block of the majority of the facial nerve fibers must begin immediately after the entrance to the fallopian channel. Only in 2 cases of idiopathic facial palsy (1 and 5) and 2 cases of herpes oticus (1 and 3) could a very small part of facial nerve fibers be stimulated from the internal acoustic meatus (stimulation site 4).

Between the stimulation sites 1 and 2 (1 mm distal and proximal to the geniculate ganglion) only a slight decrease of amplitude could be observed at most. This does not mean, however, that block of impulse conduction in part of the nerve fibers begins

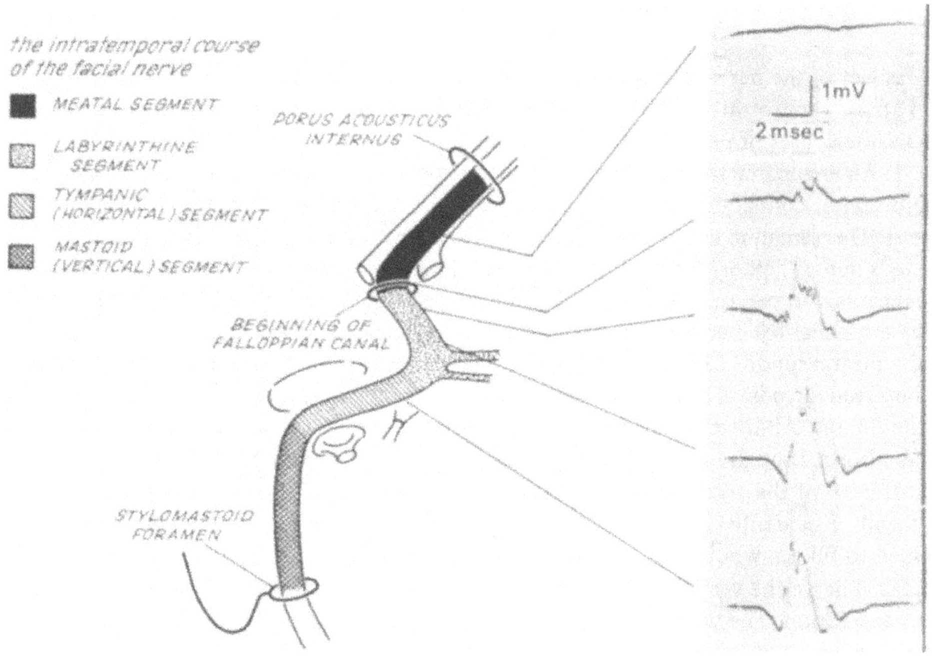

Fig. 4. Intratemporal stimulation of facial nerve

in this segment. One must take into account that nerve degeneration proceeds in distal direction from the site of damage. When the "front of degeneration" of a part of the nerve fibers has just reached the level of the geniculate ganglion, a sudden decrease of amplitude will occur when the nerve is stimulated immediately proximal to the "front of degeneration". This sudden shift of amplitude could simulate a conduction block.

2. The latencies or differences of latency between the single sites of stimulation were very constant in each case, but the comparison within the group of all cases does not reveal a systematic, regular behavior in relation to duration and severity of the nerve lesion. This may be partly due to the differences in distance between the sites of stimulation in different individuals.

3. Comparing the swelling of the nerve and its strangulation at the entrance to its canal one could be in doubt as to which of the two phenomena is more impressive, but one must consider the one as a correlate of the other. The electrophysiologic findings prove that the site of strangulation of the nerve is decisive for the functional disturbance. The close correspondence between morphologic and electrophysiologic findings in idiopathic facial palsy, herpes oticus, and Melkersson Rosenthal syndrome must be emphasized.

Table 2.1 Intratemporal stimulation of facial nerve and morphologic aspect of nerve in transtemporal decompression. Idiopathic facial palsy

No.	Patient	Date of operation	Number of days after palsy onset	Latency msec	Amplitude μV	Aspect of nerve through operation microscope
1	M. M. 23 y. f.	20. 6. 70	9	1) 4.0 2) 4.6 3) 8.0 4)	1.250 1.100 120 0	Dura in int. audit. can. opaque. Hemorrhages and engorgement of nerve in meatal fundus. Strangulation at the entrance of fallop. can. Injected vessels in labyrinthine segment until genic. ggl. After splitting of nerve sheath protrusion of nerve over the lumen of bony can. Normal aspect distal of genic. ggl.
2	E. M. 44 y. m.	24. 11. 70	9	1) 6.1 2) 6.8 3) 7.2 4)	1.000 950 450 0	Increased injection of dura vessels throughout int. audit. can. Hemorrhages and gross swelling of nerve in the fundus. Strangulation at entrance of fallop. can. Injected vessels in labyrinthine segment. No abnormality distal of genic. ggl.
3	L. M. 41 y. m. case 80	14. 6. 71	8	1) 4.2 2) 4.5 3) 5.0 4)	1.700 1.500 350 0	Reddish color of dura in int. audit. can. Hemorrhage and gross swelling of nerve in the meatal fundus. Compression of vestib. nerve by swollen facial nerve. Severe strangulation at entry to fac. can. Hemorrhage of labyrinthine segment. Distal of genic. ggl. nothing abnormal.
4	G. A. 47 y. m. case 117	23. 3. 72	7	1) 6.0 2) 7.0 3) 9.8 4) 10.8	1.350 1.350 750 100	Hemorrhage and swelling in meatal fundus. Compression of vestib. nerve by engorged fac. nerve. Severe strangulation at entry to facial can. Injected vessels of labyrinthine segment. No abnormality distal of genic ggl.
5	A. V. 23 y. m.	31. 10. 72	9	1) 9.2 2) 9.7 3) 10.1 4)	150 140 20 0	Severe hemorrhage and swelling in distal segment of int. audit. can. Vestib. nerve not inspectable due to engorgement of fac. nerve. Severe strangulation at entry to fac. can. Injected vessels in labyrinthine seg. Nothing abnormal distal of genic ggl.

Table 2.1. (continued)

No.	Patient	Date of operation	Number of days after palsy onset	Latency msec	Amplitude μV	Aspect of nerve through operation microscope
6	H. F. 34 y. m. case 131	28. 5. 73	6	1) 4.5 2) 4.8 3) 6.1 4)	460 440 180 0	Gross swelling of nerve in meatal fund (ϕ twice that of labyrinthine seg.) Engorged fac. nerve pushes vestib. nerve aside. Strangulation at entry to fac. can. Injected vessels in labyrinthine seg. No abnormality distal of genic. ggl.
7	Y. B. 42 y. f. case 140	13. 6. 73	5	1) 9.6 2) 10.2 3) 10.4 4)	280 200 40 0	Hemorrhage and gross swelling of nerve throughout int. audit. can. Strangulation at entry to fac. can. Reddish color. of labyrinthine seg. No abnormality distal of genic ggl.

Table 2.2 Intratemporal stimulation of facial nerve and morphologic aspect of nerve in transtemporal decompression. Herpes oticus

No.	Patient	Date of operation	Number of days after palsy onset	Latency msec	Amplitude μV	Aspect of nerve through operation microscope
1	E. P. 46 y. m. case Z10	2. 5. 71	8	1) 4.0 2) 4.8 3) 6.0 4) 7.6	1.150 1.150 250 40	Three quarters of the meatal segment of fac. n. show hemorrhage and gross edema. Vestib. nerve pushed aside and anemic. Strangulation at entry of fac. can. No abnormality of labyrinthine segment and beyond.
2	O. L. 57 y. f. case Z4	29. 10. 71	4	1) 4.2 2) 4.8 3) 5.0 4)	800 800 300 0	Hemorrhage and swelling greater part of meatal segment. Strangulation at entry to fac. can. Injected vessels of labyrinthine seg. Protrusion of nerve after slitting of sheath over the lumen of the canal. Nothing abnormal distal of genic. ggl.

Table 2.2. (continued)

No.	Patient	Date of operation	Number of days after palsy onset	Latency msec	Amplitude μV	Aspect of nerve through operation microscope
3	M. H. 55 y. m. case Z8	22. 12. 71	2	1) 4.0 2) 4.3 3) 4.8 4) 5.0	1.150 1.150 700 230	Hemorrhage and severe edema throughout int. audit. can., maximal in fundus. Severe strangulation at entry to fac. can. Reddish color. of labyrinthine seg. Normal aspect distal of genic. ggl.
4	V. R. 42 y. m. case Z3	10. 8. 72	7	1) 2) 3) 4)	1.700 1.100 350 0	Hemorrhage and gross swelling in the audit. can. so that vestib. n. no longer identifiable. Strangulation at entry to fac. can. Further distal no abnormality.
5	G. H. 61 y. f. case Z16	31. 3. 73	9	no measurement as nerve degen. already complete		Very conspicuous swelling and hemorrhage in fundus. Upper branch of vestib. n. is compressed. Strangulation at entry to fac. can. Hemorrhage in labyrinthine seg. Beyond that no abnormality.
6	I. H. 21 y. f. case Z14	10. 3. 73	8	no stimulation		Balloonlike engorgement of fac. nerve in meatal fundus. Severe hemorrhage. On lifting the released fac. nerve the compressed upper branch of vestib. nerve becomes visible. Strangulation at entry to fac. can. Distal of genic. ggl. no abnormality.
7	B. Z. 31 y. m. case Z17	21. 3. 74	9	no measurement as nerve degen. already complete		Hemorrhage and edema of nerve in meatal fundus. Pronounced strangulation at entry to fac. can. Edema as well of labyrinthine segment and upper part of tympanic segment. Therefore opening of the whole fac. can. No abnormality in distal part of tympanic nor in mastoidal segment.
8	U. W. 28 y. m. case Z12	17. 5. 74	8	No stimul.		Enormous swelling and hemorrhage of nerve in meatal fundus. ϕ 3 times that of labyrinthine seg. Severe strangulation at entry to fac. can. Reddish color. of labyrinthine seg. down to genic. ggl. Beyond no abnormality.
9	B. L. 19 y. m. case Z19	24. 2. 71	28	No stimul.		Edema of genic. ggl. and pronounced swelling of major superfic. petrosal nerve.

Table 2.3 Intratemporal stimulation of facial nerve and morphologic aspect of nerve in transtemporal decompression. Melkersson-Rosenthal-syndrome

No.	Patient	Date of operation	Number of days after palsy onset	Latency msec	Amplitude μV	Aspect of nerve through operation microscope
1	D. D. 24 y. m.	5. 12. 69	10	1) 5.2 2) 6.4 3) 6.8 4) 12.0	1.500 1.350 500 100	Hemorrhage and edema of nerve in meatal fundus. Strangulation at entry to fac. can. Increased injection of vessels in labyrinthine seg. of facial nerve as well as of maj. superfic. petrosal nerve. Nothing abnormal distal of genic. ggl.
2	E. P. 40 y. m case V3	13. 12. 72	33	no measurement		Dilatation of epineural vessels in fundus of int. audit. can. as well as in the labyrinthine segment of fac. nerve. After slitting of epineurium inflation of nerve to twice of its initial circumference. Normal condition of genic. ggl. and distal nerve segment.

2.2. Findings in Favor of a Revised Conception of the Relevant Pathogenetic Factors in Acute Facial Palsies

2.2.1. Histopathologic Findings in Idiopathic Facial Palsy (Table 2.4.)

As idiopathic facial palsy is not a lethal disease, it is not remarkable that histopathologic investigations are rare. During the last 83 years, only 6 cases have been published. The patients died of other diseases some weeks to months after onset of idiopathic facial palsy but at autopsy special attention was paid to the facial nerve.

In some publications one finds other cases included (Darkschewitsch and Tichonow, 1893; Flatau, 1896; André-Thomas, 1907). Reading the original communications one realizes that these cases represent either symptomatic facial palsies or palsies temporally related so closely to herpes infection that they cannot reliably be distinguished from herpes oticus. Even the famous case of Déjerine and Theohard (1897) apparently belongs to this group, as the manifestation of facial palsy was preceded some weeks to not more than 2 months before by a zoster infection in the area of the cervical plexus. Déjerine himself supposed this connection and confused Bell's palsy with herpes oticus by talking of a "rheumatic" facial palsy caused by a herpes infection.

The question is, how representative the 5 cases are. On examining Table 2.4 one realizes that only a single case, that of Fowler, has been examined early enough after onset of palsy for there to be a chance of finding the changes in the acute phase of nerve disease. It will be shown in the second part of this monograph that according to the evidence of electrophysiologic investigations the acute phase of the nerve affection does not last for more than 10 days in over 90% of the cases and for the rest not longer than 12 days. The acute phase is immediately followed by the phase of recovery and restitution. Therefore even the case of Alexander, autopsied on the 26th day of palsy, cannot be considered as representative of the acute phase. Fowler's case shows some remarkable particularities in comparison to the other 4 cases: "Most striking and unexpected were the fresh hemorrhages in and around the facial nerve in the internal acoustic meatus between the region of the normal vestibular ganglion (Scarpa's) and the narrow bony channel of the porous acousticus proximal to the geniculate ganglion. Here there were several quite large and separate intraneural hemorrhages as well as general infiltration of the nerve with red blood cells ... No evidence of inflammation of any kind was found. There was nerve degeneration in the region but this was not complete."

Fowler found some nerve swelling and extravasates of erythrocytes also in the more distal segments of the fallopian channel. The alterations, however, that he observed proximal to the geniculate ganglion were far more impressive, inducing him to express repeatedly surprise and astonishment: "For an ardent advocate of fallopian canal decompression in facial paralysis, ... the finding of pathologic changes in the seventh nerve proximal to the geniculate ganglion ... was at first *a bit disquieting*."

Fowler, himself an adherent of the theory of ischemia in the distal segment of the facial canal as the pathogenetic basis of Bell's palsy, could not believe what did not fit into this concept: "... the hemorrhages were almost undoubtedly fresher than two weeks, that is, there is considerable question as to whether they were concerned in the production of the facial paralysis."

Table 2.4 Histopathologic findings in idiopathic facial palsy

Author Year of publication	Patient Sex	 Age	Duration of palsy before autopsy	Histopathologic findings
1) Minkowski, 1891	m.	27 y.	8 weeks	Degeneration of facial nerve distal of genic. ggl., most pronounced in the peripheral nerve branches. No inflammatory signs. Interpret. of author: Pure "degenerative neuritis".
2) Déjerine and Theohari, 1897	f.	81 y.	4 months (?)	Facial nucleus: Chromatolysis. Eccentric displacement of nuclei. Facial nerve: Within the fac. can. degeneration of moderate number of fibers. Chorda tympani: Some degenerated fibers. Peripheral facial nerve branches: Degen. of the major. of fibers. No signs of inflammation. Interpret. of author: "Rheumatic" facial palsy by herpes zoster infection.
3) Alexander, 1902	m.	27 y.	26 days	Complete degeneration distally from genic. ggl., partial degen. of the segment immediately proximal of genic ggl. Complete degen. of maj. superfic. petrosal nerve. No cellular infiltrates in epi- and perineurium but numerous in endoneurium. Interpretation of author: "Peripheral neuritis".
4) Miralllié, 1906	m.	76 y.	39 days	Facial nucleus: Swelling of nuclei, chromatolysis in most motoneurons. Facial nerve: Degen. of part of the fibers. No signs of compression (no exact localisatory indications). Peripheral nerve branches: Most fibers are degenerated. Interpretation of author: "Peripheral neuritis".
5) Fowler, 1963	m.	60 y.	14 days	Fresh hemorrhages of facial nerve in meatal fundus. Small intraneural hemorrhages within the fallop. can. Engorged veins. No signs of inflammation. Degeneration of the majority of fibers distal of entry to fac. can. Interpretation of author: Causal relation of hemorrhage with facial palsy is doubted. The case is considered "unique".

Table 2.4. (continued)

Author Year of publication	Patient Sex	 Age	Duration of palsy before autopsy	Histopathologic findings
6) Proctor, B. D. A. Corgill, G. Proud 1976	m.	44 y.	14 days	"Swelling of nerve trunk in internal meatus and limited swelling of nerve trunk as it passes through temporal bone proximal to geniculate ganglion. Axons, ganglion cells and myelin are beginning to swell." "Within the facial nerve phagocytosis of myelin by macrophages, lymphocytic infiltration throughout the entire course of the facial nerve from the internal auditory meatus to the stylomastoid foramen." "Acute inflammatory changes in the nerve trunk with subsequent swelling and compression of the vascular channels in the fallopian canal."

Thus, he gives a remarkable example of how a kind of ideologic fixation by a concept, never sufficiently substantiated by empirical facts, prevents insight into the real context of the observed phenomena. He noted the differences between his observations and the generally recognized concept, but the decisive idea did not come to him, that he had found the true site of the nerve lesion due to the short time delay between death and histopathologic examination.

There is a striking conformity between Fowler's finding and our observations of the facial nerve under the operative microscope, listed in Table 2.1. His illustrations prove, though he does not expressly mention it, that the hemorrhagic and grossly swollen facial nerve is reduced to approximately one half of its diameter at the entrance to its canal. The nerve on the healthy side, which is also depicted by Fowler, does not fill out the entrance to the fallopian canal, no doubt because of some shrinkage due to fixation. But it does tightly fill the canal at the site of the palsy.

Fowler's communication is very important. because he describes what cannot be seen through the operative microscope: the *intraneural* hemorrhagia, the congested veins, and the diminution of these changes toward the distal segment. These findings could serve as a basis for agreement with those who insist that the essential pathogenetic processes occur distally to the geniculate ganglion. What appears to those, who dispose of the technique of transtemporal exposure of the acoustic meatus and the fallopian channel, as remote effects of the decisive processes, seems to be the principal finding to those to whom only the distal segments of the fallopian channel are accessible.

Just as this monograph was going to press, the author learned of the communication of Proctor et al., published in the Transactions of the American Acad. Ophtal. and Laryngology. This would be the sixth case of autopsy of an idiopathic facial palsy (if it is "idiopathic" facial palsy). The patient was a 44-year-old Negro who was admitted to hospital at the 3rd day after onset of palsy. On the 11th day he was taken to the operating room for facial nerve decompression. Twenty minutes after intubation, before any incision, he had cardiac arrest. Though external cardiac massage was instituted immediately and spontaneous cardiac activity is said to have restarted 3 minutes after arrest, the patient did not regain consciousness and died 3 days later, that is, the 14th day after onset of palsy. This accident is perhaps not surprising as blood pressure on admission to hospital was 230/130 mm Hg and autopsy revealed myocardial hypertrophy, coronary atherosclerosis, hepatomegaly, arteriolar nephrosclerosis and old and recent cerebral infarcts.

The pathologic findings differ in two important aspects from the other cases of idiopatic facial palsy: 1) Acute inflammatory changes in the nerve trunk as well as in the chorda tympani. 2) Signs of Wallerian degeneration "throughout the entire course of the facial nerve from the internal auditory meatus to the stylomastoid foramen." The authors themselves believe that the inflammation of the nerve may well be due to viral disease and relate it to an infection with Epstein-Barr virus (Grose et al., 1975). Though the authors present 10 figures of microscopic sections one would have liked to have this important case more thoroughly documented. The most proximal view of the nerve, hematoxylin x10, shows approximately 5 mm of the facial nerve in the internal auditory canal, its entry to the fallopian canal and the labyrinthine section onto the geniculate ganglion. This segment is described as follows: "Note swelling of nerve trunk in internal meatus and limited swelling of nerve trunk as it passes through temporal bone proximal to geniculate ganglion." The section presented shows very well the swelling of the nerve in the fundus and the sudden reduction of its diameter to less than one half, but, perhaps due to low magnification it is not possible to recognize Wallerian degeneration of the nerve in the internal meatus itself. The authors do not compare their case to other findings at autopsy in idiopathic facial palsy as well as in zoster oticus nor do they discuss the impact of their findings. There is no indication of any examination of cerebrospinal fluid nor of the state of the nerve in the cerebello-pontine angle or its intrabulbar course and its nucleus. Obviously, the histopathologic changes of this case would fit better to the picture known from zoster oticus. Apart from the slight cellular infiltrations in Alexander's case nobody else has ever seen conspicuous signs of inflammation in Bell's palsy. On presenting the illustrations to a neuropathologist for evaluation he considered the "inflammatory" signs as "non-specific" and possibly a cellular reaction to degenerating and phagocytised myelin sheaths (Prof. Ulrich, Basle, personal communication). Therefore a final judgement is hardly possible and it would be worthwile to reexamine the whole material, to indicate exactly at what level Wallerian degeneration starts, and what other changes may be due to reactions of nerve tissue not necessarily leading to degeneration etc. As long as this is not done the title of the communication "the pathology of Bell's palsy" appears to be rather pretentious.

Biopsy

To the post-mortem findings just mentioned can be added some histologic observations from biopsies. Some authors took advantage of the opportunity provided in "decompression" of facial nerve in the mastoidal segment. In most cases, pieces of the epineurium or perineurium, of the geniculate ganglion, or chorda tympani were taken (Jongkees, 1954, 1957; Kellel, 1959; Miehlke, 1959, 1973; Sade et al., 1965). The findings were not very revealing. No inflammatory alterations could be found, nor anomalies of the vessels. The findings are not very representative, because the material was taken from an inappropriate site, and too much time had elapsed since onset of palsy (e.g., Miehlke, 1959, 9 weeks).

2.2.2. Histopathologic Findings in Herpes Oticus (Table 2.5.)

Among the nonsymptomatic and nontraumatic facial palsies, the one occurring together with herpes oticus is practically the only one with proved viral etiology. The spread of the virus, as well as the factors determining local manifestation of pathologic processes, are still unsolved puzzles. Also the sequence of the particular pathogenetic processes has not been cleared up sufficiently.

In contrast to the six autopsy cases of idiopathic facial palsy, nine cases of herpes oticus verified by autopsy have been published. Again, each of these cases is not equally representative. Special interest must be paid to those with a relatively short latency between manifestation of disease and autopsy, i.e., cases 7 and 8. Case 3 is especially informative because of the detailed description of the findings on peripheral nerves, spinal cord, and brain. Case 2, on the contrary, can be considered only with reserve, because here herpes oticus was complicated by purulent otitis on both sides and periarteritis nodosa. The significance of cases 4 and 9 is very much limited by the long latency between onset of the zoster eruptions, facial palsy, and autopsy. Close examination of case 8, one of the two with the shortest latencies, reveals that it is not truly significant. There was only slight facial palsy, improving as early as the 3rd and 4th day, and histologic examination showed only small neuritic signs of the 7th cranial nerve. The principal changes were situated at the trigeminal nerve including its ganglion and nuclei

From the nine communications represented in Table 2.5, the following conclusions can be drawn:

1. In every case, more or less pronounced changes of "neuritis" of the 7th cranial nerve can be found (eventually other cranial nerves are likewise affected).

2. An affection of the geniculate ganglion, contrary to the assumption of Hunt, is by no means obligatory. In two cases (3 and 5) no pathologic changes could be found at the geniculate ganglion. In five other cases the pathologic findings were insignificant. Only in case 8 could severe changes be observed.

3. Few authors mention explicitly the findings in the area of the facial nucleus. Here either no pathologic changes could be found (case 8) or they were only slight, in the form of an axonal reaction (case 3).

4. One must be well aware of the distinction between the extension of the pathologic findings to different regions of the peripheral and central nervous system and the clinically relevant changes. Many authors, following Denny-Brown et al. (1944), have interpreted herpes oticus as a manifestation of a meningomyeloencephalitis, because these authors described inflammatory and degenerative changes in the peripheral nerve, spinal ganglion, spinal cord, and brain stem. It is, of course, justifiable to talk in this sense of a meningomyeloencephalitis. One should keep in mind, however, that facial palsy in herpes oticus is by no means the consequence of an encephalitis, even if some of the cases show some perivascular infiltrates in the brain stem. By no means have all of these caused symptoms during lifetime. The functional disturbance of the facial nerve is obviously a consequence of a "neuritic" process, initiated by a more or less profuse hemorrhage in the nerve itself. It is remarkable that the only significant "early" case (case 7) shows profuse hemorrhages of the facial nerve between pons and geniculate ganglion, which have led to severe destruction of nerve fibers. This histopathologic finding has to be correlated with our nine operated cases (see Table 2.2), all representing "early" cases with the exception of case 9. In the final stage, when blood extravasates have been resorbed, infiltrates of lymphocytes and plasma cells prevail, together with more or less pronounced nerve fiber degeneration.

Integrating the histopathologic findings and the experience gained on operated cases one must conclude that in herpes oticus with facial palsy the nerve is directly affected. An encephalomyelitis may cause additional symptoms, though in our series of 21 patients there were no signs suggestive of such a complication.

It is possible, however, that the statement "no facial palsy in herpes oticus without *direct* (viral) affection of the facial nerve" must be made more specific. What Ramsay Hunt assumed to be the general rule, i.e., the primary affection of the geniculate ganglion, affecting secondarily the facial nerve by edema, pressure, and consequent ischemia, may exceptionally occur. In our case 9 (Table 2.2) the principal finding was swelling of the geniculate ganglion and, particularly pronounced, in the major superficial petrosal nerve. This patient, however, happened to be the only "late" case in our case histories of operated patients. Only two authors deal with the problem of hemorrhages, which, according to our experience, dominate the initial phase of the affection of the nerve. Grünberg (1961, case 7) states: "In our case the main findings caused by zoster infection are extravasates of erythrocytes whilst cell infiltrates are inconspicuous. The same holds for the system of semicircular canals and the mucosa of tympanic cave." As Grünberg could not know the operative findings, he considered the possibility of an agonal genesis of the extravasates of erythrocytes, but dismissed this idea after taking into account the presence of phagocytized red blood cells.

Denny-Brown et al. (1944), too, touch on the problem of hemorrhage: "Hemorrhages into the ganglion, when present, appear to arise from small vessels in the necrotic region" (p. 228). On page 227 they write: "The total destruction of the body of the dorsal root ganglion closely resembled infarct necrosis." Thus, the basic idea of the authors seems to be (although they do not say so explicitly), that the primary event, as far as the hemorrhages in an encephalomalacic focus are concerned, would be necrosis of a whole region including parenchyma, connective tissue, and vessels, with secondary rupture of the necrotic walls of the vessels. However, "the large vessels, both arterial and venous, which lay outside the ganglion were of normal appearance." This statement indicates that at least the necrosis of the ganglion could not have been primarily caused by ischemia, as happens in an encephalomalacic focus.

Another strong argument against the concept that necrosis precedes hemorrhagia is the fact that some of the facial nerve fibers preserve their capacity for impulse conduction for days or even longer. Maintaining the analogy of the hemorrhages in encephalomalacic foci, one should expect a delay of days until the occurrence of hemorrhages. The course of events, as can be followed up clinically and electrophysiologically, refutes this idea. It would be out of the question to find even the remains of impulse conduction, if the severe hemorrhages of the nerve to be seen with the aid of the operative microscope were to indicate a necrosis of this nerve segment of some days duration.

The time course of events, i.e., the joint occurrence of hemorrhages and maintenance of sometimes even considerable remains of nerve function suggests that the processes elicited by the viral attack on the nerve either primarily affect the walls of the vessels, especially the endothelium of capillaries, or, if all tissue components of the nerve are simultaneously affected, the reaction of the capillary endothelium may be the most precipitated. Evaluating all known facts, we must emphasize the statement that hemorrhages of the nerve in herpes oticus cannot result from a preceding necrosis of the nerve but must be due to a primary reaction of the vessels.

Finally the question should be discussed as to why the case of Grünberg, corresponding so well to our operated cases with respect to the temporal conditions, did not likewise show a maximum of swelling of facial nerve in the fundus and the corresponding strangulation at the entrance to the fallopian canal. The argument could be that this simply escaped the author, that he did not consider this possibility. Another explanation may be more obvious, taking into account the duration of the interval between death and fixation of tissues for histologic examination. With the cessation of arterial pressure there is no longer a force effective in maintaining the vicious circle at the entrance to the facial canal. On the contrary, almost passive physical processes tend to a gradual drainage of the extravasations in proximal and distal direction. If, therefore, fixation of tissues is not performed soon after death, it could be possible that the equalization of pressure and liquid has advanced so far as to mask swelling and strangulation to a certain extent.

Table 2.5. Histopathologic findings

No.	Author	Patient Sex	Age	Duration from manifestation of herpes eruptions to autopsy	Site of herpes eruptions	Duration of facial palsy before autopsy	Facial nerve	Facial nucleus	Geniculate ganglion	Particularities, additional findings
1	Ramsay Hunt 1907	m.	48 y	87 days	Auricle, occipital, and cervical region	87 days	Lymph cell infiltrates in vicinity of geniculate ganglion	Not examined	Not examined	Necrosis of 3rd spinal ganglion, partial degeneration of 1st and 2nd spinal ganglion
2	Maybaum and Druss	m.	51 y	Some weeks	Tympanum, ext. meatus auricle	Some weeks	Uncharacteristic nerve fiber degeneration vicinity of geniculate ganglion	Not examined	Not examined	Case complicated by periarteritis nodosa and purulent inflammation of middle ear
3	Denny-Brown et al.	m.	62 y	64 days	Ext. meatus C1–C2	53 days	Lymph cell infiltrates, scattered over the whole nerve. Nerve within fallopian canal only slightly affected, considerably more the proxim. segment	Chromatolysis of some motoneurous (axonal reaction)	Normal	Necrosis of 2nd cervical ganglion and complete degeneration of its nerve. Infiltration of lymphocytes in anterior root C2 and in the corresponding medullary segment. Medulla obl.: Some small infiltrates of lymphocytes
4	Findlay 1952	m.	52 y	3 months	Ext. meatus, auricle		Some lymph and plasma cells scattered over the whole nerve	Not examined	Some lymphocytes and plasma cells. Degenerations of some motoneurons.	

Table 2.5. Histopathologic findings (continued)

No.	Author	Patient Sex	Age	Duration from manifestation of herpes eruptions to autopsy	Site of herpes eruptions	Duration of facial palsy before autopsy	Facial nerve	Facial nucleus	Geniculate ganglion	Particularities, additional findings
5	Sachs and House 1956	m.	70 y	14 months	Ext. meatus and auricle	14 months	Lymphocytes and plasma cells prox. and dist. of geniculate ganglion	Very slight axonal reaction	Normal	
6	Guldberg Möller et al.	f.	78 y	6 weeks	Ext. meatus, auricle	6 weeks	Infiltration of lymphocytes, considerable nerve fiber degeneration. No intraneural hemorrhages	Not examined	Some lymphocytes. "Slightly" degenerative cells	
7	Grünberg 1061	f.	68 y	8 days	Ext. meatus Cavum conchae, palate	8 days	Severe alterations between pons and geniculate ganglion less so distal of geniculate ganglion. Hemorrhages with severe destruction of nerve fiber structure. Infiltrates of lymphocytes and monocytes.	Not examined	Slight hyperemia of small vessels. No cell changes, no infiltrates	Cochlear and vestibular nerve are also affected (clinically hearing difficulty and spont. nyst.). Rather slight perivascular hemorrhages and small cell infiltrates in the vicinity of nerve sheath. Hyperemia and hemorrhages also in the "effector organ" (mucosa of mastoid cells and tympanic cave).

Table 2.5. Histopathologic findings (continued)

No.	Author	Patient Sex	Age	Duration from manifestation of herpes eruptions to autopsy	Site of herpes eruptions	Duration of facial palsy before autopsy	Facial nerve	Facial nucleus	Geniculate ganglion	Particularities additional findings
8	Bethlem 1962	f.	76 y	4 weeks	Ext. meatus, left face and tongue	4–5 days	Some round cell infiltrates, scattered over the nerve	No changes	Round cell infiltrates, severe cell alterations but no necrosis	Partial necrosis of Gasserian ganglion. Numerous round cell infiltrates in Gasserian ganglion and trigeminal nerve. Severe affection also of the cells of trig. nucl. Round cell infiltrates in the "effector organ" (tongue)
9	Blackley et al. 1967	f.	69 y	30 weeks	Auricle	30 weeks	Profuse infiltrates, frequent perivascular along the whole petrosal course. Demyelination	Not examined	Very few cells show vacuolization and atrophy.	1. Cochlear nerve in internal auditory canal: Hemorrhages and some infiltrates of lymphocytes. Axons generally intact. 2. Spiral ganglion: Considerable perivascular round cell infiltration. 3. Vestibular nerve Scarpa's ganglion: Gross hermorrhages, infiltration of lymphocytes. 4. Labyrinth: Some perivascular round cell infiltration vicinity of macula. 5. Middle ear: Perivascular infiltration of lymphocytes and plasma cells in mastoid cells.

2.2.3. Integration of Morphologic and Electrophysiologic Findings

The previous exposition permits the following statements:

1. The morphologic findings with the aid of the operative microscope after exposure of the internal acoustic meatus and the proximal segment of facial canal are practically identical in idiopathic facial palsy and in herpes oticus. Perhaps in herpes oticus, hemorrhagia and swelling of the nerve are even more pronounced than in idiopathic facial palsy, but this quantitative difference of rather statistical character would not permit a distinction in the individual case when one is dealing with herpes oticus or idiopathic facial palsy.

2. The electrophysiologic findings are likewise identical. Conduction block is localized in both conditions at the entrance to the facial canal.

3. Morphologic as well as electrophysiologic findings prove that in both diseases the pathogenetically relevant processes occur at the entrance to the facial canal. The alterations, occasionally to be observed on more distal segments of the nerve are nothing but remote effects.

So much correspondence provoke the question as to the differences between the two conditions. The previous statements prove, not the identity of both diseases, but the fact that, beyond a certain point, the pathogenetically relevant processes apparently correspond in both conditions to an astonishing degree. As will be shown in Section 3.4.4, the whole acute phase of both nerve diseases is characterized by this correspondence. In both diseases the phase of nerve fiber degeneration is terminated not later than the 10th–12th day. Apart from this correspondence, somewhat conducive to the postulation of a viral etiology for idiopathic facial palsy, too, definite differences can also be formulated:

1. In herpes oticus extensive perivascular infiltrates of lymphocytes are a regular finding, frequently outlasting the acute phase of the disease by months. In idiopathic facial palsy, on the contrary, all authors stress the absence of inflammatory signs, with the single exception of Alexander (1902), and Proctor et al., 1976 (cf. p. 28) who observed numerous cellular infiltrates in the endoneurium, but not in the peri- and epineurium. Because of the scarcity of histopathologic findings one must be careful to accept the described difference as complete and total.

2. In idiopathic facial palsy the vestibular and cochlear nerves are not affected, while in herpes oticus this complication is rather common. The slight functional disturbance described by Lämmli and Fisch (1974) and Robert and Pfaltz (1970), which can be demonstrated in the electronystagmogram, is caused, in our opinion, by the pressure exerted on this nerve by the swollen facial nerve. Even in herpes oticus the more severe affection of the vestibular nerve may be partially due to its compression by the facial nerve (see 3.4.3). Some strangulation of the nerve is clearly visible under the operative microscope. It would be an exaggeration, however, to ascribe the whole extent of vestibular (and cochlear) disturbance to the compression of these nerves by the swollen facial nerve. The histologic examination of these nerves has revealed hemorrhages and infiltrates of lymphocytes, though much less pronounced than in the facial nerve (see Table 2.5, Nos. 7, 9).

3. In zoster oticus, severe damage to the facial nerve is far more frequent than in idopathic facial palsy. Out of 21 cases of zoster oticus, 11 (= 52%) showed complete

degeneration of the nerve, whereas in 145 cases of idiopathic facial palsy only 9 (= 6%) nerves degenerated completely.

4. In zoster oticus, different parts of the peripheral and central nervous system may be affected; in idiopathic facial palsy only the nerve is affected.

Impressive as the correspondence of a part of the pathogenetic processes may be, the difference between the two conditions cannot be disregarded. What, then, are the final conclusions?

1. The hitherto prevailing concept on the localization of the pathogenetically relevant processes in the distal segment of the fallopian canal must be abandoned in view of the evidence showing the maximal affection of the nerve at the entrance to the facial canal.

2. If two etiologically different nerve affections show the same morphologic and functional changes at the entrance to the facial canal, it must be assumed that local factors determine a great part of the pathogenetically relevant processes.

3. If zoster oticus, to date never explained in terms of *primary* and *secondary* ischemia, shows hemorrhage, strangulation, and impulse conduction block in the same way and at the same site as idiopathic facial palsy, it must not be assumed that primary ischemia is a precondition of the latter. Then the hypothesis of the initial vasospasm, which was to explain primary ischemia, would be superfluous.

What, then, could replace primary ischemia? The example of zoster oticus answers this question. Vasodilation and hemorrhage, which can already be observed on the second day with the operative microscope, have not originated the same day. They certainly existed the day before, with great probability even before manifestation of the palsy. These are the same changes shown by cases of early histopathologic examination. All evidence, therefore, indicates that the first recognizable vascular reaction in zoster oticus is not vasoconstriction but dilatation and a severe disturbance of permeability, leading to extravasation of red blood cells. Why should not this be the first vascular reaction in idiopathic facial palsy, too, to a noxa, the nature of which, admittedly, is still unknown?

The next link in the chain of pathogenetically relevant events can be easily deduced. As hemorrhage and edema of the nerve in the fundus of the acoustic meatus cannot continue into the facial canal, they must cause its strangulation at the entrance to its proper canal. Here, at this site, not only the epineural blood supply is blocked, but also the intraneural microcirculation breaks down. At this point local ischemia of the nerve arises. This ischemia at first blocks impulse conduction of the nerve fibers, but with longer duration more and more nerve fibers will be damaged to such a degree that Wallerian degeneration follows. The damage to the connective tissue, increasing with the duration of ischemia, must also be taken into account, as its condition is of eminent importance for regeneration.

This revised concept of pathogenesis will not solve all problems. However, it does make the sequence of pathogenetic events more comprehensible. The hypothesis of the primary and secondary ischemia may very aptly explain the "vicious circle": primary ischemia followed by intraneural edema, which causes increase of intraneural pressure leading to secondary ischemia and blocking of venous and lymphatic drainage. One of the questions, vainly put in this context, was how this vicious circle could be stopped, which, once initiated somewhere in the facial canal, caused necrosis of the whole nerve segment in the fallopian canal. For this pathomechanism must have possessed a kind of self-propagating effect, inevitably contaminating the neighboring nerve segments. If, however, the edema of the nerve causing local strangulation is at the entrance to its canal, no self-propagating vicious circle is initiated, but strangulation will cease with the remission of the vascular reaction. The edema can easily be drained off in the direction of the acoustic pore.

The crucial point of the revised pathogenetic concept presented here is the relation of the "local" to the "general" factor. The latter causes the primary disease of the nerve. This primary disease preferentially affects the proximal segment, according to the evidence exposed in this monograph–morphologic aspect under operation microscope, conduction block with intraoperative nerve stimulation and late onset of conspicuous slowing of impulse conduction in the distal segment (see 3.4.2.3).

This primary disease, causing vasodilation and swelling, would not have serious consequences if the facial nerve did not have to enter and pass a long narrow bony canal. Without a fallopian canal, Bell's palsy would probably be a rare disease and herpes oticus far less severe.

Whatever agent causes swelling of the nerve in the internal auditory canal, be it a direct viral attack or a vascular reaction to a sensitizing noxa, the sudden transition of the swollen nerve to a narrow canal, allowing no extension, must cause strangulation at this site. It may well be that with a *short* narrow pass as, for instance, the foramen ovale for the 3rd trigeminal branch, there would be some drainage of the nerve in distal direction, but the length of the fallopian canal prevents such relief.

Thus the local factor can be clearly denominated: narrowness and length of the passage through the fallopian canal. This local factor is operative in all types of non-bacterial acute facial palsies, hence the striking similarity of so many parameters of their natural history, as will be discussed in the second part of this monograph.

Acute facial palsy is more like a syndrome than a specific disease.

3. Investigations, Part II: Electrophysiologic Investigations on the Natural History of Acute Facial Palsies

3.1. Electrodiagnosis of the Facial Nerve

1. *General Considerations*

Electrodiagnosis should provide information as *early* and as comprehensively as possible on the state of the diseased nerve and the muscles it supplies. Each of the methods described below involves a particular routine, but none is really fool-proof. Obtaining reliable values of measurement is a matter of experience as well as interpretation. The single measurement has to be evaluated against the background of the typical reactions of the diseased nerve and the normal course of a nerve lesion. The more the diagnostician knows already, the more revealing the measurement will be.

Proximal to the geniculate ganglion the facial nerve consists of approximately 10000–12000 nerve fibers (Blinker and Glaser 1958; van Buskirk, 1945: cf. 1.1.2). Approximately 7000 are myelinated motor fibers, the rest sensory and vegetative fibers, partly myelinated, partly nonmyelinated. As will be seen later, only the state of the motor fibers can be evaluated by electrodiagnosis with sufficient reliability.

As long as a nerve lesion does not lead to immediate destruction of the tissue, a graduated reaction of the nerve fiber population is to be expected, i.e., a spectrum of reactions. These nerve fiber reactions have a morphologic and a functional aspect. Both aspects must be combined for the definition of a nerve lesion.

The function of nerve fibers is impulse conduction, nothing else. In respect to this function two degrees of nerve fiber lesion can be distinguished: (1) slowing of impulse conduction, (2) block of impulse conduction. Frequently, in these stages of nerve lesion no morphologic changes can be observed on the axon and on the myelin sheath, especially where the functional disturbance is of short duration. With longer duration alterations on Schwann cells and myelin sheath are detectable, and segmental demyelination in particular. The third stage of nerve lesion is characterized by abolition of impulse conduction in Wallerian degeneration of the nerve fiber but no damage to the connective tissue, especially the endoneurium. In the fourth stage damage to the connective tissue is added to Wallerian degeneration. In the fifth stage there is complete rupture of the nerve.

Each of these stages has its particular implications. Slowing and block of impulse conduction may be reversible states or transitions to degeneration. Thus, the presence of impulse block does not indicate by itself the *direction* of the process. The definition of stages 3 and 4 takes into account not only the functional and morphologic state of the single nerve fiber but also the condition of the connective tissue. The importance of the condition of the connective tissue is generally underestimated. All components of the connective tissue must be taken into account, the endoneurium enclosing the single nerve fiber, the perineurium surrounding the fascicle of nerve fibers, as well as the epineurium sheathing the whole nerve. Electrodiagnostic long-term prognosis of a nerve palsy is not possible without consideration of these conditions. Integrity of the endoneurium is far more important for good recovery of nerve function than occurrence or absence of Wallerian degeneration. Intact endoneural tubes practically always guarantee good recovery, as the regenerating axons find a preformed guide-rail, leading them to their original site of innervation. Serious damage to the endoneurium prevents regeneration of nerve fibers. The consequence is formation of intraneural scars, barring the way of the axon sprouts to the periphery. The axons may be successful in getting around such obstacles but do not find their way back along their proper endoneural tubes. Instead, they follow whatever tube they find to the periphery. This misdirection of the regenerating nerve fibers is not of great consequence as long as a regeneration nerve supplies a muscle or muscle group of uniform function, as for instance the musculocutaneous nerve. If, however, the muscles supplied by a nerve have very different functions, as is the case with the facial muscles (and those innervated by the ulnar nerve or the oculomotor nerve) the regenerating nerve fibers may be directed to a "wrong" muscle—for instance to the orbicular muscle of the eye instead of the oral muscles. As the central (supranuclear) patterns of mimic and reflex-innervation cannot be reprogrammed, the consequence of such a misdirection of regenerating axons must be an inappropriate activation of certain muscles, while the muscles originally innervated by the now misdirected fibers are likewise reinnervated by "foreign" fibers or receive no fibers at all, thus remaining paretic (cf. 3.4.2.6).

The proper task of electrodiagnosis is to provide a statistical assessment of the general condition of the nerve. The first objective is to establish the relation of blocked to degenerated nerve fibers. The aim should be to indicate this relation as an exact percentage. As will be shown in the following section only electroneurography (supramaximal stimulation of the nerve—recording of the compound action potential with surface electrode) can fulfill this requirement in facial palsy.

The second objective should be to establish the *direction* of the process. For this purpose generally several control measurements are required which should be performed at optimal time intervals.

2. *Special Problems of Electrodiagnosis of the Facial Nerve*

In contrast to most lesions of peripheral nerves, electrodiagnosis of cranial nerves is hampered by one big difficulty. In the majority of cases it is not possible to stimulate proximally to the site of the lesion. Thus, it is not possible to compare the response on proximal stimulation with the response on stimulation distally from the site of the lesion. But such a comparison is essential for the determination of the relation of blocked to degenerated nerve fibers. The same holds for the precise *localization* of the site of the lesion, which is not difficult in spinal nerves, as long as it is not situated too near to the nerve root. The most unfavorable conditions are encountered in electrodiagnosis of eye muscle nerves, because here it is not even possible to stimulate the peripheral nerve section in a manner acceptable for clinical routine. Stimulation proximal to the site of the lesion, which would be the ideal diagnostic procedure, is possible only in exceptional cases, i.e., at operation. Thus, any electrodiagnostic method which is to be regularly performed on facial nerves must base its conclusions on the result of stimulation only in the short segment between the stylomastoid foramen and the point where it starts to branch off. Therefore, the quantitative determination of the relation of blocked to degenerated fibers depends on finding another point of reference. Before presenting the solution of this problem, a survey of the electrodiagnostic methods applied up till now will be given.

3. *Electrodiagnostic Methods Hitherto Applied for Diagnosis in Facial Palsy*

Nerve and muscle are both electrically excitable though with different thresholds. By adequate combination of the so-called parameters of stimulation, i.e., *duration* and *strength* of the electrical impulse, it is possible to conclude from the effect of stimulation if the muscle or muscle group is supplied by a functionally intact or disturbed nerve. In the classical method of electrical diagnosis, the minimally perceptible muscle twitch serves as indicator. Therefore, with this method, stimulation is always in the range of threshold of the most excitable nerve or muscle fibers. However, in modern diagnosis by nerve stimulation with square wave impulse combined with the recording of the compound action potential (electroneurography), maximal or even supra-maximal stimulation is required to guarantee the discharge of all excitable fibers.

On stimulation with increasing impulse strength (duration and amplitude of the impulse are the effective parameters), the nerve fibers will discharge on lower impulse strength than muscle fibers. Muscle twitch, provoked by nerve stimulation, is called indirect excitation. In direct excitation the denervated muscle fibers discharge directly, without the bias over the nerve. Due to the high utilization time of the muscle, direct stimulation is only possible either with direct current (the old galvanic stimulation) or with square wave impulses of sufficient duration–not less than 10 ms, and preferably 30 ms. Today, direct excitability of the muscle is of importance only in two cases: (1) In plotting the strength-duration curve of a denervated muscle; (2) if, after a prolonged duration of denervation, the question arises whether sthere is still excitable muscle tissue which could be reinnervated, for instance, by nerve transplantation. Whereas in the first case the minimal muscle twitch on threshold stimulation serves as indicator, one must try, in the second case, to elicit the maximal muscle contraction, for only in this way it is possible to estimate the amount of muscle tissue which still may be reinnervated.

Diagnosis by electrical impulse is in a state of transition. The older methods of stimulation with the minimal perceptible muscle twitch as indicator (chronaxy strength-duration curve, and excitability test) are rapidly giving way to electroneurography. Nevertheless, these older methods will be briefly reviewed here, because many clinics, especially in otology, do not yet have the new methods and equipment, nor the trained staff.

1. *Strength-Duration Curve.* First, the rheobase must be determined, i.e., the current strength eliciting a just perceptible muscle twitch when sufficiently sustained. In this technique the duration of current flow is of importance. In denervated muscle one must start with a duration of 300 ms. With intact nerves, the threshold is practically constant between 0.3–0.1 s. Therefore, in this range, the strength-duration curve of the nerve runs parallel to the abscissa and rises steeply with shorter impulse duration. The strength-duration curve of denervated muscle shows a pronounced rise already with an impulse duration of 100 ms. In comparison to the strength-duration curve of the nerve it shifts considerably toward the right side. Regenerating muscles show an intermediate strength-duration curve. In partially denervated muscles without regeneration the curve is not very indicative. In fact only in severe denervation is there a significant upward shift.

The plotting of a complete strength-duration curve is a rather time-consuming procedure. Attempts have been made therefore, to reduce it to a determination of one significant point on the curve, defined by specific parameters. The following two procedures have been derived from the strength-duration curve: chronaximetry and the excitability test.

2. In *chronaximetry* the chronaxy is determined, i.e., the impulse duration that provokes just perceptible muscle twitch with a current of twice the strength of rheobase.

3. More important for electrodiagnosis of the facial nerve is the *excitability test* (Laumans, 1965). In this procedure the current strength (in mA) is determined which elicits a just perceptible muscle twitch when applied during a previously defined time. The method of determination of impulse duration is a little imprecise. The majority of authors agreed to apply an impulse of 0.3 ms duration (Richardson, Wynn-Parry, Laumans, Jongkees). Thus, in the excitability test the only variable is current strength.

In normal persons a considerable range of threshold values has been found (2.4–16.2 mA according to Jongkees; 6.5 mA according to Laumans). On the other hand threshold differs but little between the two facial nerves of one individual. Therefore, the value on the healthy side has been taken as reference. According to Jongkes the mean difference of threshold intensity between both sites is 0.4 mA (SD 0.2 mA).

A difference of 3.5 mA is considered to be pathologic. If the difference can be observed during the first days of a facial palsy, control measurements can indicate the direction of the process. Increase of threshold on the affected side indicates increase of degeneration of nerve fibers.

For the adherents of an operative procedure the question is to know at what value an intervention is indicated. On this point, however, there is no reliable information available in the literature. This lack of precision is not surprising if we remember that in the excitability test measured values are not clearly correlated to a precisely defined functional state of the nerve. This holds true even for the value "infinite" which should indicate complete degeneration of all nerve fibers. In some patients, where no muscle twitch is perceptible on electrical stimulation of the facial nerve, single active motor units can be observed in the EMG or even a compound action potential of low amplitude may be recorded. As will be seen later, it is of great importance for prognosis to know whether the facial nerve has totally degenerated or whether individual nerve fibers have been preserved. In the first case one must assume that strangulation of the nerve at the entrance to the fallopian canal has been so strong as to cause Wallerian degeneration of all fibers and equally severe damage of the connective tissue, whereas in the second case, with preservation of some nerve fibers, damage to the connective tissue will be less severe.

We have examined the reliability of the excitability test together with our own method which indicates the degree of degeneration of the facial nerve directly as a percentage. It was shown that the degree of degeneration, when the excitability test becomes "significant", varied between 60 and 90%. Thus, we do not believe that the excitability test is useful for early prognosis, the precondition for the indication of an operative intervention.

4. In some places the so-called *maximal excitability test* is applied (May, 1976). In this method stimulus strength is maximal in order to bring all nerve fibers that are still excitable to discharge. The strength of the muscle twitch provoked in this way is estimated simply by clinical observation. There is no recording or plotting. With some experience this test gives earlier and more reliable information than the excitability test, but it is not possible to determine precisely enough the relation of blocked to degener-

ated nerve fibers. In cases of subtotal degeneration both tests are practically identical.

5. *Latency.* In 1965 Taverner published an investigation of 167 patients with "spontaneous" facial palsy in which the latency between the electric stimulation of the nerve and the response of the muscle was taken as an indicator for the degree of damage the nerve had suffered. The author states: "The prognosis in spontaneous facial palsy can be reliably established in the first few days by studying the conduction time in the facial nerve branches in response to percutaneous electrical stimulation. Patients developing complete denervation of the facial muscles lose all response to percutaneous electrical stimulation. Patients developing complete denervation of the facial muscles lose all response to electrical stimulation after 5 days from paralysis."

We have included in our investigations latency in most of the patients. Our results do not confirm the statement of Taverner: Latency proved to be a rather slow and unreliable indicator for the evaluation of the damage the nerve had suffered. Furthermore, it happens only in very rare cases that degeneration is already complete by the 5th day of palsy (cf. 3.4.2.1).

6. *Electromyography and Electroneurography.* Originally electromyography signified the recording of motor unit potentials in voluntary and involuntary muscle contractions and of spontaneous activity of the muscle fibers as, for instance, in denervation. Very soon, however, this elementary electromyography was supplemented by the recording of the compound action potential, elicited by the supramaximal stimulation of the nerve. In order to distinguish this method from the original electromyography it has been named electroneurography.

Simple electromyography is not very revealing in facial palsy of recent origin. Without stimulating the nerve it cannot be decided if loss of innervation is due to conduction block or to degeneration of nerve fibers. The so-called denervation potentials can be recorded only after 8 to 10 days, and frequently even later. They are only a qualitative indicator of denervation but do not reveal whether it is complete or partial. Therefore, Kaeser and Pfaltz (1963) have thus qualified the value of electromyographic investigations: "In idiopathic facial palsy, prognosis cannot be sufficiently substantiated by electromyography before the end of the 4th week."

Nevertheless, two important findings ought to be mentioned, where EMG can be very helpful: (1) As long as a few active motor units can be recorded, even if there is no visible contraction of muscle fibers at all, the lesion of the facial nerve has not yet reached the point of severe degeneration and if this lasts until the 7th day of palsy, severe degeneration will not occur. (2) If, after a period of complete arrest of all motor unit activity some units resume discharging, this signals onset of recovery from conduction block even days before any visible muscle contraction. If this happens up to the 15th day of facial palsy, prognosis is good.

4. A New Method for the Determination of the Degree of Degeneration of Facial Nerve

Comparison of the amplitude of the compound action potential in supramaximal stimulation of the facial nerve on both sides in healthy persons has shown that there is very little difference. In a group of 30 healthy persons the mean difference in amplitude was 3%. In half the persons practically identical values were measured on both sides. In some persons differences up to 5% were found and one showed a difference of 8%. On the basis of these results it appears justifiable to take the compound action potential of the facial nerve on the healthy side as reference, and to represent the amplitude on the paretic side in percent of the amplitude of the normal side. Thus, the value obtained in this way represents the percentage of fibers still excitable though blocked for impulse conduction. The difference in this value when compared to the healthy side indicates the percentage of fibers already degenerated.

This way of indicating the degree of the nerve affection is a statistical statement of the state of the facial nerve, i.e. of the relation of fibers that are only blocked to degenerated fibers. When we consider that the facial nerve contains approximately 7000 motor fibers it is evident that only such statistical statements are relevant.

The Compound Action Potential (Figs. 5 and 6). The compound action potential is the result of the synchronous discharge of motor units. In the normal case, when all fibers of a nerve are stimulated to the point of discharge, the corresponding motor units will discharge, too. To assure the discharge of all excitable fibers one must apply "supramaximal" shocks, i.e., one has to increase stimulus strength approximately 20% over the strength just sufficient to discharge all nerve fibers. The "maximal" impulse strength, just discharging all nerve fibers, is very variable in different persons. It depends on the resistance of the skin, and the thickness of tissue between stimulating electrode and nerve. In contrast to the excitability test, however, stimulus strength in this method has no diagnostic significance. The point is to stimulate supramaximally.

The potentials of excited nerve or muscle fibers recorded extracellularly spread according to the law of volume conduction (Rosenfalck, 1957). The amplitude of the compound action potential is proportional to the number of discharging elements, in

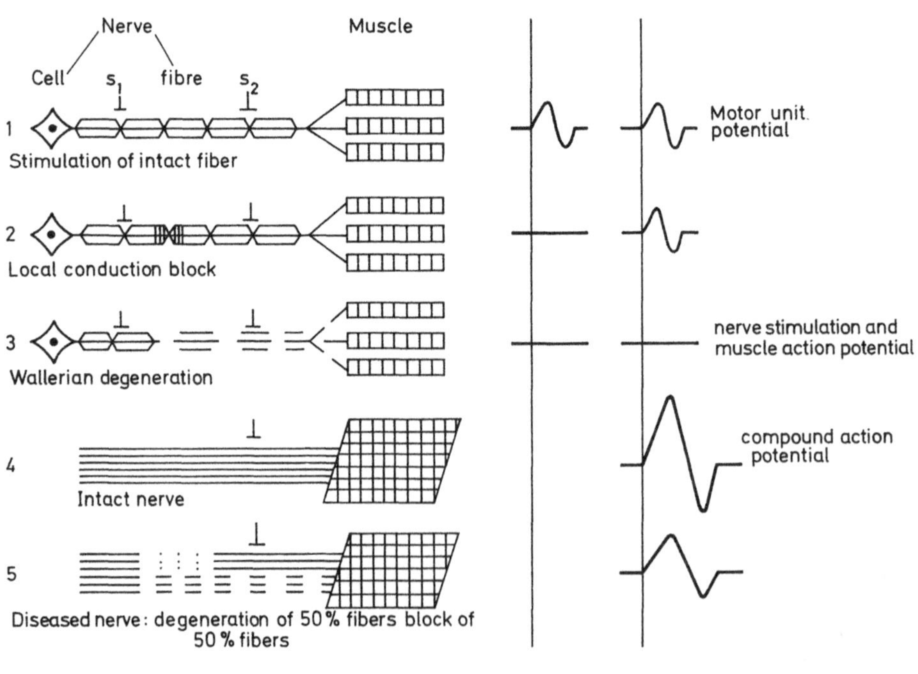

Fig. 5. Nerve stimulation and muscle action potential

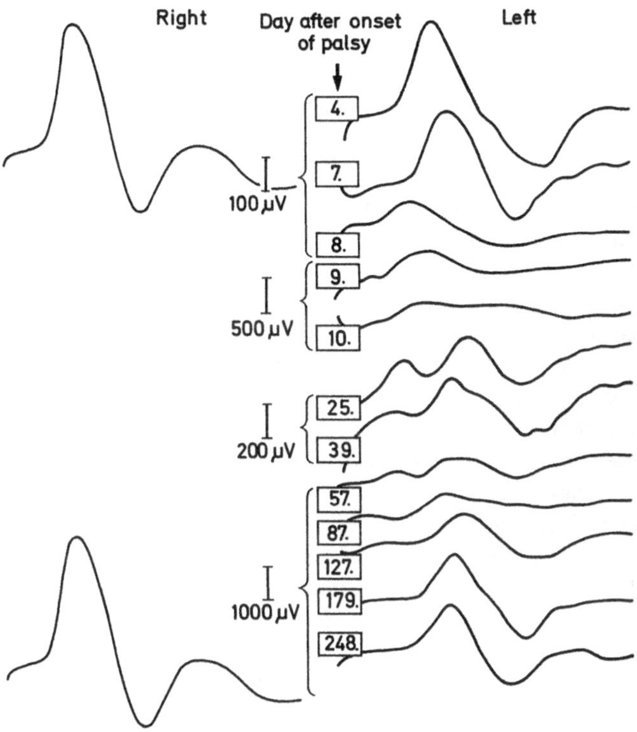

Fig. 6. Sequence of compound action potentials of paretic side (*left*) compared to the CAP of healthy side (*right*). Note that amplification is 2 x from 8th–10th day and increased 5 x from 25th–39th day of palsy

our case to the number of discharging muscle fibers. The number of excited muscle fibers is correlated to the number of motor units. Degeneration of a nerve fiber always means denervation of all the muscle fibers belonging to the motor unit supplied by the nerve fiber. The facial muscle motor units are composed of approximately 20–30 muscle fibers. The decrease of the amplitude of the compound action potential in nerve fiber degeneration is therefore proportional to the number of denervated motor units.

The shape of the compound action potential is strongly influenced by the direction of the recording electrode in respect to the course of the muscle fibers. Placing the electrode alongside the nasolabial fold, it is not too difficult to get a clear-cut diphasic or only slightly triphasic potential. In our arrangement of electrodes the first deflection was always positive (see Fig. 6), but the polarity of the first deplection is a matter of convention. The electrodes could also be placed so that the first deflection is negative. For the sake of good reproduction one should, however, always record with the same polarity.

Equipment. Basic requirements are an EMG amplifier, a display and a recording unit. Most producers will offer this as module system. We have used Medelec equipment because fiber optic recording on direct print papers offers the great advantage of having the records immediately available for measurement of amplitude, etc., without any delay due to darkroom processing.

Amplitude of Compound Action Potential. The mean amplitude on the *healthy* side of the 145 cases of idiopathic facial palsy evaluated in this investigations was 5326 μV (SD 1175 μV). The 29 male patients of this group (62.7%) showed a mean amplitude of 5432 μV (SD 1164 μV) and the female patients (37.3%) a mean amplitude of 5222 μV (SD 1248 μV).

Technical Details of the Methods. As it is not possible to record the compound action potential of *all* motor units of facial muscles simultaneously, it was necessary to find a site to record a representative number. It is legitimate in statistics to derive one's conclusions not from the investigations of all elements but from a representative part. After some trials, the recording of the perioral muscles proved to be most convenient. It would have been possible to record in addition the compound action potentials of the periorbital and frontal muscles. This would however be more time-consuming, and would probably affect the cooperation of a good many patients. It is important to choose a technique that will be tolerated in repeated investigations over periods of months. The method described here may cause some slight discomfort according to individual sensitivity, but is applicable even in the case of a child.

Recording Technique. It is absolutely necessary to record with surface electrodes to get reproducible measurements. Recording with coaxial needle electrodes is quite impracticable because even slight shifts of the needle position cause considerable changes of amplitude and latency, especially in facial muscles. It would not be possible to find precisely the same recording site again with needle electrodes.

The distance of the recording electrodes must be absolutely constant, therefore the common adhesive electrodes are not applicable. The recording electrodes must be fitted in a block of plastic material.

It is of great importance for control measurements to localize the recording site precisely. Fortunately, such an exact localization is easily possible in facial muscles, as the facial structure offers a convenient landmark for orientation. The most convenient site for this purpose proved to be the nasolabial fold, with the superior electrode placed just beside the end of the nose.

The recording with surface electrodes was preceded by a simple exploration with needle electrodes in all cases of apparently complete loss of muscle innervation. This exploration with the coaxial needle electrode serves for a quick orientation. As will be seen later it is of some importance for prognosis, depending on the time that has elapsed since onset of palsy, whether single motor units can be voluntarily activated or not. During the first 10 critical days the voluntary activation of two or three motor units not visible by clinical inspection, signifies that conduction block is not complete and therefore degeneration of nerve fibers has not yet reaches a critical level. After the 12th day the voluntary activation of a few motor units indicates that at least some fibers have survived, though degeneration may be nearly complete. In cases where the compound action potential recorded by surface electrodes is completely abolished, thus indicating complete degeneration of all motor nerve fibers, the absence of motor unit activity verified by the electrode provides an additional check.

Technique of Stimulation. The facial nerve was stimulated transcutaneously by bipolar surface electrodes as near as possible to the stylomastoid foramen, i.e., immediately below the auricle between the jaw and mastoid process. We used Disa surface electrodes with a diameter of 7 mm per electrode and a distance of 15 mm between two electrodes. Supramaximal square wave impulses of 0.2 ms duration were applied.

The rate of stimulation was 1/s. As there is an increase of amplitude in many cases during the first stimulations only the compound action potentials following the 20th stimulus were accepted for measurement. This initial increase of amplitude is probably due to two effects: (1) a decrease of skin resistance with the repetition of stimulation, (2) an improved synchronization of the motor unit potentials composing the compound action potential.

The skin under the stimulating and recording electrode should be gently rubbed with emery paper. Thus stimulus strength can be reduced as well as the stimulus artifact.

Reproducibility of Measurements. The method just described is technically rather simple. It must be stressed, however, that reliable values will be obtained only after considerable practice. Fixing stimulating and recording electrodes with adhesive tape is not recommended. There are mainly two difficulties opposing optimal recording, which can be overcome only with experience: (1) Stimulation and recording with surface electrodes causes a relatively strong stimulus artifact. Very slight alterations in respect to the direction of the electrodes or to the pressure applied to them can eliminate the stimulus artifact. (2) In the beginning it is difficult to record a compound action potential always with the same phase. We have chosen the beginning of upward deflection from zero line (in our equipment upward deflection means positivity). The compound action potential should always be recorded from the same starting point of upward deflection to ensure good reproducibility. This can be done by minute shifts of electrodes. The *simultaneous* optimal positioning of stimulation and recording electrodes requires some practice. It must be admitted, however, that the requirements for exactness in routine work may be less strict than those applied for these investigations, as in daily clinical work a deviation from the correct value up to 10% could be tolerated. For the purpose of this investigation we attained a range of 3%. This signifies with a mean amplitude for the compound action potential of 5500 μV an admissible error of measurements of 150 μV. With a range of deviation of 5% which is still acceptable for a biological method of measurement, the error could be up to 250 μV.

One should keep in mind that a range of error of 3% does not mean that the compound action potential of, e.g., 100 μV must be measured with a deviation not greater than 3 μV. As the compound action potential on the paretic side is always indicated in percent of the potential of the healthy side and this value remains constant, the value of the admissible error is also constant. A potential of 100 μV on the paretic side corresponds to 2% of the assumed normal value of 5500 μV on the healthy side. An error in the range of 100 μV would change the result only for 2%. But an error of this order is not at all to be expected. A compound action potential of the order of 100 μV can be recorded with an error of no more than 20 or 10 μV. In this case the error is in fact 10–20% of the recorded potential but the effective error is not related to the recorded potential on the paretic side but to the one on the healthy side. Under these circumstances an error of 20 μV is in fact less than 1%. This means that the range of error tends to decrease toward lower amplitudes on the paretic side. It is possible, therefore, in cases of great decrease of amplitude on the paretic side, to indicate degrees of degeneration of 97 or 98% without becoming unrealistic.

It is equally feasible to determine the point of transition from the degeneration of almost all facial nerve fibers to total degeneration.

3.2. Remarks on Some Clinical Features of Acute Facial Palsies

It is not the intention of this publication to contribute to the clinical symptomatology of facial palsies. On this subject the comprehensive reviews of Zülch (1970) and Miehlke (1973) may be consulted. Furthermore, the clinical symptoms of individual cases are not described because of space limitations. (An exception has been made, however, for the bilateral facial palsies to enable the reader to make his own judgement of the indicated diagnosis in this group. Similarly the clinical features are briefly indicated in herpes oticus and in facial palsy of different etiologies.)

Some particular points, however, will be discussed before presenting the case reports, because they contribute to a better understanding of the cause of facial palsy. When does facial palsy begin or, more precisely, when does the pathologic process leading to idiopathic facial palsy begin? When does it end?

Onset may be very abrupt. A patient with no pathologic signs in the evening may rise the next morning with complete facial palsy. In such a case the beginning of the palsy can be established quite precisely. On the other hand a patient often cannot say exactly when his palsy began. He realizes that there is a disturbance only when gross deficiencies occur, e.g., when the soup flows out of the paralyzed corner of his mouth. At that point he will systematically test the functioning of all his facial muscles, look at a mirror and discover the weakness of all the muscles of the one side of his face. Now he remembers perhaps, that he had difficulty in whistling the day before, or that he could not close the one eye when aiming at a target and so on. Sometimes the patient only realizes that there is a disturbance when somebody else calls his attention to the asymmetry of his face.

The palsy represents the clinical manifestation of the disease but not its real onset. Certain symptoms may precede the onset of palsy by several days as, for instance, intra- and periauricular neuralgias. Other precursors are burning pain in one or even both eyes, increased lacrimation, twitches of the eyelids, or dysesthesia of the upper lip and cheek. Some patients notice hyperacusis or a disturbance of taste. All these signs are of interest, not because they are indicative in respect to prognosis, as some authors believe (a point refuted convincingly by Larens [1955]), but because they help to determine the time when the sequence of pathologic processes begin. They must already have been operative at least as far back as the earliest pathological signs and de facto, of course, even longer. This question will be taken up again in the discussion of the evidence of the electrophysiologically established "profiles".

Where is the point of termination of the disease? When there is complete recovery of palsy? Or, in the case of defective recovery, could the end be dated from the time when no further improvement is detectable? There is, as in other diseases, no simple answer to this question. Concerning facial palsy one can state in general: The disease has terminated when the pathogenetic processes causing the functional disturbance of the nerve are no longer effective. What criteria could be named to serve for orientation? On the basis of more clinical observation of the development of the disease it would make sense to fix the termination of the disease at that point of the time axis when recovery from axon block is detectable (rise of "palsy curve"–now preferably called "recovery curve"). Recovery from axon block is only possible when the pathogenetically relevant factors are no longer operative. There is another feasible time mark to indicate termination of the disease which is based on the electrophysiologic investigations exposed in this monograph: the day when nerve fiber degeneration comes to a standstill. There may be some overlap of both time indices in slight and medium cases. In cases of severe palsy, however, nerve fiber degeneration always comes to an end before recovery from axon block. This point will be further discussed in a later section, also (cf. 3.4.2).

We should like to propose that the following phases of the course of the disease be distinguished: (1) The acute phase of the nerve lesion. This lasts from the beginning of the first symptoms, including the so-called prodromal signs or preceding symptoms, until the end of degeneration of the nerve fibers. This time point can be established by electrophysiologic methods. (2) The restitutive or recovery phase. This has two sections: a) recovery from block b) regeneration of nerve fibers and/or reinnervation of facial muscles.

In assessing the functional result at the end, the clinical observations should be correlated with, and integrated into, the underlying neurophysiologic and pathologic processes. The first step towards recovery is the return of facial symmetry. If such symmetry is attained by all the mimetic and other functions of the facial muscles, recovery will be clinically complete. For the patient this is what matters most. However, if we look at the problem from the biological and/or pathophysiologic aspects, then in many cases even complete return of the facial symmetry is far from indicating complete recovery of the facial nerve. As will be discussed in more detail in a later section (3.4.2.4), observation alone will not suffice to detect a loss of up to 40 or 50% of facial nerve fibers, provided that impulse conduction by the remainder continues intact.

But sometimes it is the other way around: although the electrophysiologic investigation shows that a relatively high number of fibers have regenerated, mimetic function continues to be poor. This is almost always the case when there is marked associated movement and facial contracture. These phenomena can be attributed to misdirection by the regenerating axon sprouts. This kind of misdirection always occurs when the connective tissue, and particularly the endoneurium, is also severely damaged and the endoneural tubes are lacerated, causing intraneural scarring. The regenerating axons cannot find the way back to their own tubes, and take false directions through others, which lead to connections to "wrong" muscles. Fibers which previously innervated the M. orbicularis oculi may thus connect to a perioral muscle, or vice versa (see also Esslen 1960, Fisch and Esslen 1968). This aspect will also be more fully discussed in a later section (cf. 3.4.2.6).

3.2.1. Implications of Topical Diagnosis

It is part of the established technique for the neurologist and the otologist to test the functioning of the parasympathetic (n. petrosus superficialis major) and sensory (chorda tympani) nerves which branch off from the main nerve in the facial canal, and to seek to deduce the site of the lesion from the result of such investigation. Thus a disturbance of lacrimal and salivary secretion points to a lesion above the exit of the n. petrosus superficialis major, while a disturbance of the sense of taste indicates a location above the exit of the chorda tympani. Such a diagnostic investigation will also include the motor nerve branching off between the parasympathetic and sensory nerves to the stapedius muscle, which, if affected can lead to hyperacusis. Tschiassn (1953) has gone furthest with this kind of topical diagnosis, but many other authors consider its value in practice to be rather limited. This is not the place to argue the matter. There is a more fundamental aspect of the question which should be examined in the present context, and which until now has received little attention.

Specific tests have been developed to demonstrate malfunctions of the lacrimal and salivary secretions, the sense of taste, and the stapedius muscle reflex. Originally considered as essentially qualitative, these tests have been progressively refined to yield quantitative data, e.g. the Schirmer test, the salivation test, the measurement of the stapedius muscle reflex, and electrogustometry. As each of these quantifying procedures has evolved, it has been accompanied by increasingly confident assertions concerning its value in prognosis. Such claims have been made with particular insistence in the last few years in regard to the salivation test and electrogustometry.

But two issues have to be kept in mind: (1) The question whether, for example, taste fibers have been affected by a lesion of the facial nerve or not depends not only on the level of the damage but also on the extent of the lesion in relation to nerve cross section.

A lesion of the facial nerve above the exit of the chorda tympani must not necessarily involve in relation to its cross section so many taste fibers as to cause a perceptible loss of taste.

Since it has become possible to register summation potential at the human extremities we know that a considerable number of sensible fibers must be precipitated, often in excess of 50%, before a disturbance of sensibility can be demonstrated clinically. It can be deduced that a disturbance of the sense of taste will not be detected until a great many taste fibers have stopped transmitting impulses. Thus lesions of the facial nerve which occur above the exit of the chorda tympani or another intratemporal nerve exit will not necessarily lead to a noticeable degree of disturbance of function. In fact, the topical diagnostic procedure is valueless in regard to the localization of the relevant pathogenetic events in idiopathic facial palsy.

(2) Furthermore, not only is the value of the procedure limited in regard to localization, but also in regard to prognosis. This, it must be pointed out, has nothing to do with any value judgment in regard to the quantification test per se. It is simply that the prognostic value of these tests stands or falls on whether it is possible to decide during the acute phase of the nerve lesion whether impairment of function is a result of blocked conduction of the impulse or degeneration of the nerve fibers. Since this acute phase, during which the final outcome of the lesion is in fact settled, lasts at most 10 days (see also 3.4.2, et seq.) the precise nature of the disturbance must be established whithin that time. Unfortunately, there is no way of applying these tests which can produce an answer to the question. Experience indicates that indeed the prognostic value of such tests is meager, and demonstrably so. Thus, in group 1 of our cases of idiopathic facial palsy, we included all cases in which only slight or no degeneration of the facial nerve was detectable. Three of the six patients in the group had ageusia, and every member improved within a short time.

3.3. Case Reports

From the patients available the following cases were chosen:

1. 145 bases of idiopathic facial palsy
2. 21 cases of facial paresis associated with herpes oticus
3. 8 cases of bilateral facial palsy
4. 8 cases of facial palsy of various etiologies
5. 6 cases of facial paresis caused by trauma

The main criterion for selection was the presence of a sufficient number of measurable changes, occuring in particular during the period immediately after onset of palsy. In fact it would have been desirable with regard to several of the patients to have possessed even more data than were available. To those who seek perfection in this area it must be said in our defense that it is scarcely possible to expect human beings to behave like laboratory animals. In the majority of cases, the investigations were carried out on an ambulatory basis, and therefore certain considerations, such as the age of patients, their general condition, distance from the hospital, etc., tended to influence the frequency of the examinations. The regularity of examination was also affected by events such as the absence of patients on vacation or on business, or by the occurrence of other illness. Finally, it is not easy to maintain the cooperation of patients who lead busy lives when the palsy is already more or less extinguished and therapy has in any case virtually ceased. In short, there are limits to what is possible.

A second, but important, criterion for selection in this series was that the patient should have had as short a latency as possible between the 1st day of illness and the 1st day of investigation. As can be seen from Table 3a–1, it was possible to examine 80 of the 145 patients with idiopathic facial palsy, or 55%, by at the latest the 5th day of illness, and to record the compound action potential. Such a large number of early cases must be considered as a very favorable element in the situation, particularly when one bears in mind that patients present first, not at the university clinic, but to their family doctor. He as a rule sends to the clinic only those cases which show no improvement after several weeks. It was a similar situation with regard to the herpes oticus group, in which 15 of the 21 patients, or 71%, were examined for the first time by the 7th day of illness at the latest.

The two above-mentioned criteria were not always strictly observed, however. A small number of cases were also included in which the first investigation was carried out relatively late, i.e., after the 15th day of palsy. This is worth mentioning because it shows that the information produced by the complete graph after examination can throw light on the early section of the curve as plotted.

Interesting possibilities were created by the fact that comparison could be made between the evolution of disease in a group of patients with facial palsy of known etiology but about whose pathogenesis we still have a great deal to learn (herpes oticus), and a group of patients with idiopathic facial palsy, whose etiology is unknown. This applies also to a great extent to the group with bilateral facial palsy, because it was possible to use the appropriate electrophysiologic methods of investigation to make extremely accurate comparisons of the course of the disease between one side and the other. The same considerations apply, mutatis mutandis, for the group with palsies of various other etiologies, and which in some instances are known. Finally, the study also included a small group with facial palsy of traumatic origin, following petrosal bone fracture, because of the obvious importance of finding ways of improving the possibilities of prognosis with regard to this type of injury.

The 145 cases of idiopathic facial palsy were divided into nine groups, with the extent of nerve fiber degeneration as criterion:

Group	Degeneration (%)
1	0– 10
2	10– 30
3	30– 50
4	50– 70
5	70– 90
6	90– 95
7	95– 98
8	98– 99
9	100

It can be observed that degeneration in the sector 90–100% was divided into four groups. This was because a preliminary review showed that those cases with the worst prognosis were distributed around a paresis grade of 95%. In regard to the possibility of surgical (transtemporal) decompression, it was clear that only cases in the 95–100% area of degeneration could be considered. Therefore this section was divided into three groups, so that selection criteria for possible decompression could be formulated as precisely as possible.

In the herpes oticus group the total number of cases was so small that such finely graded divisions were not feasible. In fact two groups emerged:

Group	Degeneration (%)
1	50– 95
2	95–100

The clinical signs in herpes oticus were so clear that there were practically no doubts as to the correctness of the diagnosis.

However, it would be too much to hope that similar certainty prevailed concerning the 145 cases presenting as idiopathic facial palsy. In fact it seems likely that in certain cases there was another, underlying, etiology, a mild lymphocytic meningitis, or a single-symptom polyradiculitis (compare cases VI and V2). As has been pointed out in section 2.2.3 it is doubtful, anyhow, whether idiopathic facial palsy constitutes an etiologically uniform group.

3.3.1. Discussion of the Graphical Presentation of Results

In a desire to present the data in a visual, quickly assimilable form, the compound action potentials for the affected side of the face were at first set out in chronological order, as seen in Fig. 6. However, it soon became evident that this method of presentation was time-consuming and not sufficiently concise. In consequence the method of presentation shown in Fig. 7 was adopted, which refers to the same case as Fig. 6 (cf. p. 47). This method presents the whole history at a glance, including the acute phase of the nerve lesion, recovery from conduction block, and regeneration. Furthermore, additional parameters such as latency and the degree of paresis can also be included. Some points require additional explanation, however:

1. *Time Axis*

Since in many cases the period of observation was very long (up to $3\frac{1}{2}$ years), it was not practical to seek to express the time period on a metric scale. This would mean, in particular, that the changes occurring in the acute phase would be unduly compressed, with a consequent loss of clarity. A logarithmic time scale was therefore adopted, on which the first 10 days take as much space as the following 90 days, and the 900 days after that. The time-axis dimension can also be taken as days, so that a history of up to 1000 days can be displayed on a single sheet.

The 1st day of the time axis is also the 1st day of palsy (see also section 3.3.0). It begins, not with zero, but with Value 1. An entry over the numeral 2 signifies the 2nd day of palsy, and not that 2 days have passed since the day the palsy began.

2. *Vertical Axis*

2.1. The amplitude of the compound action potentials of the affected side (*thick line*) is expressed as a percentage of the potentials of the unaffected side. The summation potential of the healthy side is thus always given a value of 100%. If for example a compound action potential of 90% is entered on the 2nd day, this means that the amplitude on the affected side is one-tenth lower than that on the healthy side. This 10% indicates the degree of degeneration of the nerve, i.e., 10% of the nerve fibers have degenerated.

The 1st day of palsy is only in a few cases the 1st day of investigation or recording of data. Much more often the 1st examination day occurred between the 1st and 6th day of palsy. Thus the thick line indicating the compound action potential is entered as discontinuous during the period from the 1st day of palsy to the 1st day of examination, and only then becomes continuous. The discontinuous line not only indicates the presumed history of degeneration in the days before the first measurement, but also what may loosely be termed the gradient of the fall in amplitude. This discontinuous line was not used if the 1st day of investigation fell after the 15th day of palsy, as in fact occurred in a small number of cases.

2.2. *Latency*. The thin line represents the latency. This was established in the majority, if not all of the cases. The latency (the time which elapses between stimulation of the facial nerve behind the angle of the jaw and the beginning of the compound action potential) can be taken directly from the graph in milliseconds (ms) if the numerals on the left of the y axis are taken as single units instead of units of 10. Thus the numeral 30 means 3.0 ms latency.

2.3. *Degree of Palsy*. Some attempt must be made to establish a relationship between the degree of palsy and the measurements of the degree of degeneration of the facial nerve. Since objective criteria for the calculation of the degree of palsy do not exist, this relationship has to be formulated on the basis of estimations. However, we can at least establish the two limiting values. The absence of any detectable sign of innervation on the affected side indicates an innervation degree of 0% or a degree of palsy of 100%. An absence of any asymmetry of the facial innervation, and no loss of innervation, represents a degree of palsy of 0%. A degree of palsy of 40% corresponds to an innervation grade of 60%. Both values are in complementary relationship to the numeral 100. For the sake of simplicity, the term "degree of palsy" was chosen and used exclusively. The 100% degree of palsy, which means complete loss of innervation or paralysis, is expressed by the zero line. No loss of innervation, or a degree of palsy of 0%, is expressed by the 100% line. To read off the degree of palsy, which is presented as the medium line on the graph, it is only necessary to subtract the numerals on the left side of the curve from 100. So 10 becomes 90, 20 becomes 80, and so on.

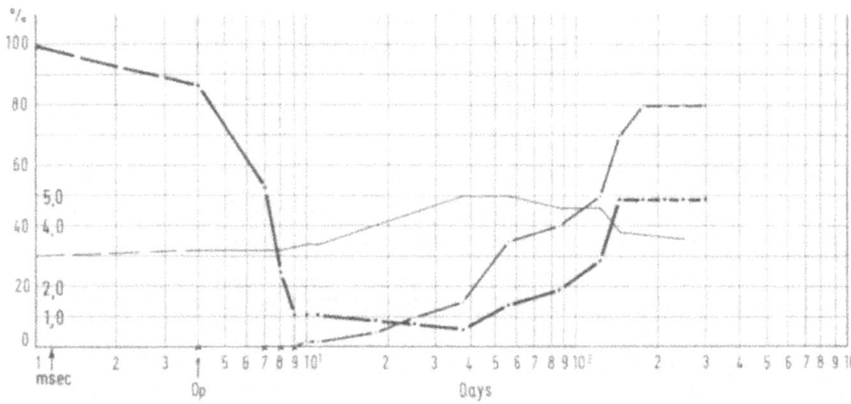

Fig. 7. Diagram presentation of natural history of facial palsy. 1. Amplitude of paretic side plotted in percent of CAP of the healthy side (*thick line*); 2. Estimated degree of facial innervation in percent (*medium line*); 3. Latency between stimulus and CAP in ms (*thin line*)

A point that might be raised here is whether it might not have been more practical to adopt the method of Jongkees, so widely followed elsewhere, in which the division is made in degrees of severity. But this cannot be expressed in percentages, is less clearly graduated, and the subjective factor which has to be introduced in making the estimations is certainly no less. It is interesting to note, incidentally, that visitors to our laboratory adapted so quickly to this method of appraisal that variations of more than 10% between physicians present were extremely rare. The fact that the technique was applied by a single investigator during the whole period offers a further assurance of consistency in the application of the criteria of appraisal.

Originally the intention was to present the diagrams of all cases included in this monograph. This, unfortunately, was not possible due to economic reasons. Because of this limitation only the diagrams of the first six patients in each group can be presented with the exception of some additional diagrams raising particular questions. All results are included, however, in the different tables.

3.4. Results

3.4.1. Idiopathic Facial Palsy (Groups 1–9)

Group 1 (0–10% degeneration)

Cases 1–6
Sex: 4 male, 2 female
Localization: 5 on right side, 1 on left.
Average age: 32 years (14–45 years)
The patients came between the 2nd and 10th day of palsy for the first investigation (see Table). In cases 1 to 4 no sign of degeneration of the facial nerve could be detected. In cases 1 and 3 the loss of innervation appeared complete for several days, although the electromyograph was always able to detect some motor unit activity. The conduction block of the facial nerve in these two cases was high, but not complete. In case 2 there was clearly a partial conduction block from the beginning. In case 4 because of the late conclusion of the first investigation the extent of maximal block could not be estimated. In cases 5 and 6 the later evolution of the graph would indicate that at the beginning conduction block was not complete.

Three of the six patients complained of early symptoms such as a burning sensation in the eyes, dysesthesia in the part of the face which later became paretic, and also on that side of the tongue. The duration of such symptoms was from 4 days to a few hours before palsy onset. Case 2, V. H., aged 42, also complained of position-dependent vertigo, which began some weeks before the onset of palsy, but which then decreased in severity as the palsy receded.

Case Notes

Case 1: the palsy was clinically complete at the 4th day of palsy, but began to decrease from the 7th day, and within 14 days had completely disappeared.
Case 3: A history very similar to case 1.
Case 6: This case shows a notable deviation from the normal course of conduction block. As a rule block disappears within the first 3–4 weeks after the onset of palsy. In this instance, although the patient, aged 14, showed virtually no sign of degeneration of the facial nerve, the regeneration of the axon block began only very slowly between the 10th and 50th days. The process of recovery from residual block was completed between the 50th and 90th days.

Group 2 (10–30% degeneration)

Cases 7–15
Sex: 6 male, 3 female
Localization: Right side in 4 cases, left in 5 cases.
Average age: 42.3 years (19–70 years).
In this group, too, where there was relatively limited degeneration, half the cases showed preliminary symptoms such as dysesthesia on the side that later became paretic, periauricular pains, and lacrimation, up to 2 days before palsy onset.

In six of the nine cases the preliminary examination was made by the 5th day of palsy. Degeneration in seven of the cases had halted by the 11th day at the latest. In cases 8 and 11 amplitude decreased 5% further after the 11th day. The beginning of recovery from axon block could be established in 8 patients by the 15th day of palsy at the latest. The latency was measured in six of the nine cases. Four of these six patients showed an extension of the latency period of from 0.4 to 1.2 ms. The maximum prolongation was reached by the 6th day.

Case Notes

Case 7: At the time of the first examination, on the 2nd day of palsy, a degeneration of the order of 10% was noted, which increased only very slightly in the next 2 days. Since the latency period had already lengthened by the 2nd day of palsy, and continued to do so until the 4th day, it can be deduced that the disease process was already affecting the facial nerve several days before the acute onset of conduction block. It can also be deduced that a certain amount of weakening of the facial muscles had already set in

1 to 2 days before it reached such a degree that it was noticed by the patient. The recovery from axon block set in between the 4th and 6th days of palsy, and was complete by the 19th day.

Case 8: The process of degeneration of about 25% of the facial nerve fibers was virtually complete by the 4th day of palsy. Recovery from conduction block began on the 3rd day. By the 23rd day only a very slight residual block could be detected. The very long interval between the penultimate (23rd day) and final examination (32nd day) resulted in an unusually slow ascent of the paresis curve. It seems most probable that recovery from conduction block was complete by the 30th day. However, one noteworthy aspect of the case was the very slight degree of nerve regeneration. Several other details of the clinical history point to the supposition that this was a rather untypical case of idiopathic palsy. The history was marked by severe neuralgia within and below the ears, which was also accompanied by dizziness and vomiting in the first days of palsy, and cold dysesthesia first on the left side of the face and then bilaterally, and also in the left arm. There was also difficulty in swallowing. These disturbances regressed in the course of a week.

Case 9: The degeneration of the facial nerve fibers followed a diphasic course in this patient. The peak of the second phase occurred between the 8th and 11th days. It was striking to note that this in no way appeared to affect the recovery of the axon block, which was clearly evident from the 8th day. This second phase of degeneration cannot therefore be ascribed to a second phase of illness. It seems more likely that what occurred was degeneration of a nerve fiber population, the extent of which had already been determined during the first phase of illness. This is supported by the consistency of the data from the latency.

Cases 12 and 14 were notable for the unexpectedly high degree of clinically detectable paresis which occurred between the 5th and 11th days, without affecting the favorable outcome.

Group 3 (30–50% degeneration)

Case 16–45
Sex: 18 male, 12 female.
Localization: 16 on right side, 14 on left.
Average age: 31.8 years (12–69 years).

In 11 of the 30 cases no preliminary symptoms were reported. The rest of the patients complained of a range of symptoms, either singly or in combination, including headache, periauricular neuralgia, burning in the eyes, dysesthesia in the region of the side of the face that later became paretic as well as the corresponding half of the tongue, increased lacrimation, and minor twitching of the eye on the side that later became affected. In one case the patient had had an episode of influenza 2 weeks before the onset of palsy.

In 18 of the 30 patients the first examinations were carried out in the period up to the 5th day of palsy. In 15 cases degeneration had halted by the 7th day, and in all patients by the 10th day (in cases 44 and 45 the end point could not be precisely established, because they came for examination on the 15th day. By that time the degeneration process had already terminated). In half the patients the beginning of axon block recovery could be recognized by the 11th day of palsy, and in all patients by the 15th day. In 23 patients the latency period was also measured. Ten patients showed a prolongation of from 0.2 to 1.2 ms. In 8 patients the weakening of impulse conduction was detectable by the 7th day. In two others it could only be established between the 10th and 16th day.

Case Notes

Case 16: The patient came for examination on the day she noticed muscle weakness on the left side of the face. The measurements indicated 15% degeneration. Paralysis was clinically complete on the 3rd day, and on the 5th day the beginning of axon block recovery could be recognized. The rest of the case history resembles that of case 7.
Case 17: Degeneration was even more noticeable in this case than in case 16, and 25% was measurable by the 1st day of palsy. The patient, a female, had symptoms of head-

Table 3a. Group 1 (numerals indicate case number)

Day of Palsy	1	2	3	4	5	6	7	8	9	10	11	12	13	14	15	16	17	18	19	20	Not measurable
1st examination day		1	2	3	5 6					4											
End of degeneration phase					5 6																
Deblocking begins							1 5		6	2 3			4								

Table 3b. Group 2

Day of Palsy	1	2	3	4	5	6	7	8	9	10	11	12	13	14	15	16	17	18	19	20	Not measurable
1st examination day		7	8	9	10 11 12	13		14												15	
End of degeneration phase				7		12		10 14	9		8 11		13								15
Deblocking begins					8	7 10			9		14				11 13	12					15

ache and ocular burning sensations 2 days before. From the graph curve it can be deduced that the disease process in the nerve had already begun at least 5–8 days before the patient first noticed the facial weakness. Another noteworthy feature of this case was that prolongation of the latency first began after the axon block had begun to recover.

Case 29: In contrast to cases 16 and 17, the process of degeneration began late and reached completion rather abruptly between the 5th and 8th days of palsy. By this time recovery of the axon block had already started. The graph indicates that strangulation of the facial nerve fibers was maximal between the 1st and 3rd days.

Group 4 (50–70% degeneration)

Cases 46–66
Sex: 10 male, 11 female
Localization: 13 on right, 8 on left side
Average age: 44.2 years (13–76 years)

Of the 21 patients 8 had no preliminary symptoms. Of the others there were 3 who reported a preceding episode of influenza. The others showed the typical range of symptoms.

In 15 of the 21 patients the first examination took place by the 6th day of illness. The process of degeneration was completed in 20 patients by the 11th day at the latest. In case 57 another "late" reduction in amplitude of barely 10% was noted between the 18th and 21st days, even though at this point in time the recovery from conduction block was already progressing well. The latency period was measured in all patients. Twelve showed a deceleration of between 0.4 and at maximum 1.0 ms. by the 10th day of palsy at the latest.

Case Notes

Case 51: The curve of the recovery phase seems to be abnormal, but this is due to the fact that only one value was obtained in the later stages.

Case 56: In this instance, as in case 55, regeneration had scarcely begun by the 100th day of palsy, but after that good progress was made.

Group 5 (70–90% degeneration)

Cases 67–100
Sex: 23 male, 11 female
Localization: 12 on right, 22 on left
Average age: 45.4 years (14–69 years)

This was the largest group numerically. Twenty-five of the 34 patients came for the first examination by the 6th day of palsy at the latest. In 20 patients the process of degeneration was complete by the 11th day at the latest. In eight further cases the time when degeneration ended could not be firmly established because of insufficient data. However, it can be deduced from the graphs that in these patients also the degeneration process came to a halt by the 11th day at the latest. Five patients showed a more marked late phase in reduction of amplitude between the 11th and 27th days of illness. The clearest example was case 84, where degeneration increased from 33% to 82% between the 11th and 27th days of illness. The history indicates an obvious diphasic process (see also section 3.4.2). The beginning of recovery of the axon block could be observed in 13 patients in the 2nd week, but in the other 21 cases it started only in the 3rd week. The latency period was measured in 30 patients. Twenty-five of them showed a prolongation up to the 12th day of palsy at the latest, ranging from a minimum of 0.3 to a maximum of 6.5 ms.

Case Notes

Cases 67–70: Of the four cases in this group, all of whom were examined on the 1st day of palsy, cases 67 and 68 already showed degeneration of from 17–23%. When these cases are compared with the two following (69, 70), the differences in gradient in the degeneration curve are very marked. In cases 69 and 70 the process of degeneration had halted between the 3rd and 10th days of palsy. On the other hand, cases 67 and 68 showed a much more protracted course, although it must be added that in case 68 the

Table 3c. Group 3 (numerals indicate case number)

Day of Palsy	1	2	3	4	5	6	7	8	9	10	11	12	13	14	15	16	17	18	19	20	Not measurable
1st examination day	16 17	18 19 20 21 22	23 24	25 26 27 28	29 30 31 32 33 34	35 36	37 38 39	40	41 42	43									45	44	
End of degeneration phase		20		21 25 28	17 30 31 32	35	27 33 34 37 38 39	22 29 36	16 18 19 23 40 41 42	24 26 43											44 45
Deblocking begins						29	17 18	16 22 25 36	20 28 35	24 31 40	38 39	27		32 42 43 44		34	26	19 30 37	21 23	41	33 45

Table 3d. Group 4

Day of Palsy	1	2	3	4	5	6	7	8	9	10	11	12	13	14	15	16	17	18	19	20	Not measurable
1st examination day			46 47 48	49 50 51 52	53 54 55	56 57 58 59 60	61 62	63		64	65 66										
End of degeneration phase						47 54	55 56 57 60 61	49 52 58	62 63	46 48 53 64	50 51 65 66		59								
Deblocking begins							51 54		63	46	55 61	56 60 62	47 53 58	49 50 57	52 65		59	48 64		66	

long interval between the 3rd and 4th examinations meant that the degeneration end point could not be established with complete accuracy. It is also worthy of comment that in cases 67 and 68 the first examination did not indicate a complete loss of innervation, whereas this was found in case 69. No systematic differentiation could be made between the patients in regard to the beginning of block recovery, and the regeneration phase was also very similar in pattern throughout. No notable differences were recorded in regard either to preliminary or accompanying symptoms. From a comparison of the different histories, it can be concluded that in cases 67 and 68, strangulation of the facial nerve set in more slowly than in cases 69 and 70.
Case 72: There was a progressive decrease in the rate of degeneration, with a late phase of 12%.
Case 80: In this case transtemporal decompression was carried out on the 8th day of illness. Postoperatively only a very limited increase in degeneration could be observed. Recovery from block evolved very quickly.
Cases 92 and 97: A striking aspect of these cases was the steep gradient of the latency period between the 11th and 14th days of palsy in one case, and the 12th to the 19th days in the other.

Group 6 (90–95% degeneration)

Cases 101–112
Sex: 8 male, 4 female
Localization: 6 on right, 6 on left.
Average age: 42.3 years (16–71 years)

Of the 12 patients, 7 presented for the first examination by the 6th day of palsy. The completion of degeneration phase was reached in eight cases on the 11th day. In cases 104, 110, 111, and 112 the completion of degeneration could not be established with complete certainty, but the graph would indicate that the decisive phase had ended by the 11th day. Cases 101, 102, 103, 105, 106, and 109 showed even after the 11th day an untypical decline in compound action potential of less than 10%, which can be attributed very probably to desynchronisation of motor unit discharges, due to unequal slowing of impulse conduction in different nerve fiver populations, and not to continued degeneration.

Only in 3 cases could the beginning of recovery from block be detected before the 15th day. In all 11 cases where the latency period was measured an increase was found.

Group 7 (95–98% degeneration)

Cases 113–127
Sex: 13 male, 2 female
Localization: 10 on right, 5 on left.
Average age: 34.7 years (12–69 years)

In 10 patients the first examination was performed by the 8th day of palsy, while 4 came for the first time on the 15th day or later. In 8 patients degeneration had terminated by the 11th day. Untypical if slight reductions in amplitude were seen after the 11th day in cases 113, 114, 120, 121, and 123 (see also the case notes for group 6). In three cases the degeneration end point could not be precisely determined, but was estimated to have occurred by approximately the 11th day (cases 122, 124, and 125).

Recovery from block did not begin in any patient before the 15th day, and in fact began much later in the majority of cases. The latency period was measured in 12 patients. In all of these there was a prolongation of from 1 to 7 ms.

Case Notes

Case 117: On the 7th day of palsy, with 93% degeneration, a transtemporal decompression was performed (cf. Table 2.1, No. 4). Postoperatively the compound action potential amplitude decreased only very slightly.

Table 3e. Group 5 (numerals indicate case number)

Day of Palsy	1	2	3	4	5	6	7	8	9	10	11	12	13	14	15	16	17	18	19	20	Not measurable
1st examination day	67 68	69 70	71 72 73 74 75 76	77 78 79 80	81 82 83 84 85 86 87	88 89 90 91	92 93	94 95	96 97	98	99	100									
End of degeneration phase						90	93	74 94 95	69 75 78 85 97	67 70 77 81 82 86	71 87 91 92 96 99 100	79 80 89	76 83 88			98	73			72 84	68
Deblocking begins							75 77	76 88	69 85	82 86	96	73 83 81			79 80 84 94	78 98	71 72 99 100	90	74 91 97	67 68 70 87 92 93 95	

Table 3f. Group 6 (numerals indicate case number)

Day of Palsy	1	2	3	4	5	6	7	8	9	10	11	12	13	14	15	16	17	18	19	20	Not measurable
1st examination day		101 102	103 104	105		106 107		108		109						110				111 112	
End of degeneration phase								101		109	102 103 108	106	104	105							107 110 111 112
Deblocking begins														101 109	103	106 108		107		102 104 105 110	111 112

Table 3g. Group 7 (numerals indicate case number)

Day of Palsy	1	2	3	4	5	6	7	8	9	10	11	12	13	14	15	16	17	18	19	20	Not measurable
1st examination day			113 114	115 116 117	118 119		120 121	122			123						124	125 126		127	
End of degeneration phase								119	113 120	114 115 121	116 117 123										118 122 124 125 126 127
Deblocking begins																	123	119		113 114 115 117 118 120 121 122 124 125 126 127	116

Group 8 (98–99% degeneration)
Cases 128–136
Sex: 5 male, 4 female
Localization: 5 right, 4 left.
Average age: 41.1 years (10–73 years)

Five of the nine patients were seen by the 7th day of illness at the latest. In five, the process of degeneration had ended by the 11th day. There were some minor reductions in amplitude but these were attributable, as in the previous groups, to the increasing desynchronization of the compound action potential. This was a result of the markedly increased deceleration of the conduction of the impulse in a few fiber groups. In two cases (132, 135) the end point of degeneration could not be precisely established because the time intervals between the measurements were too great, but on all the evidence it was located at the 10th or 11th day of palsy. Only case 134 showed a reduction in amplitude of 10% after the 16th day, which was attributable to a certain extent to the progress of nerve fiber degeneration. However, the latency period rose to over 8 ms, indicating a deceleration of conduction to about one-third of original level. In such a situation a sharply increased dispersion of the compound action potential has to be taken into account, which can cause as much as a fall of 10% in amplitude. Recovery from block did not begin in any of the patients until after the 20th day of illness. The latency was measured in all patients, and in each case prolongation was indicated, which was by as much as 16 ms in some cases.

Case Notes

Case 129: Transtemporal decompression was carried out on the 9th day of palsy.
Case 131: An operation was carried out on this patient on the first examination day, i.e., the 6th day of palsy, after diagnosis of 91% degeneration (case 6, Table 2.1).

Group 9 (100% degeneration)
Cases 137–145
Sex: 4 male, 5 female
Localization: 2 right, 7 left
Average age: 40.8 (19–72 years)

In five of the nine patients in this group the first examination was carried out at the latest by the 8th day of palsy. In cases 137–140 and 142 the end point for the degenerative phase could be precisely established, but this was not possible in case 141, and in cases 143–145. In two cases degeneration set in early (in case 138 between the 4th and 6th days, and in case 140 between the 6th and 10th days). Case 137 represented a middle point, because here the degeneration process was completed between the 11th and 15th days. In case 142 the last fibers degenerated only on the 35th day of illness, even though 99% degeneration had already been reached on the 11th day. The latency was measured in all patients and found to be much prolonged.
Case 140: Transtemporal decompression was carried out on the 6th day of palsy (case 7, Table 2.1).

3.4.2. General Principles that Emerge from the Histories of Idiopathic Facial Palsy

1. Nerve Fiber Degeneration

In 125 of the 145 cases the end point of the degeneration phase could be established with considerable accuracy. This was not feasible in the other 20 cases, either because the examinations were too widely spaced, or because the patients presented for the first examination after the 10th day of palsy, and by that time the end point of degeneration had already been passed. That this was indeed the case could be deduced a posteriori. When further examinations failed to reveal any additional decline in amplitude (e.g., case 99), it was clear that degeneration was already complete by the first examination (case 122 is another example).

Table 3h. Group 8 (numerals indicate case number)

Day of Palsy	1	2	3	4	5	6	7	8	9	10	11	12	13	14	15	16	17	18	19	20	Not measurable
1st examination day			128		129 130	131	132		133			134		135						136	
End of degeneration phase								129	130 133	128 131		134								132 135 136	
Deblocking begins																					128 129 130 131 132 133 134 135 136

Table 3i. Group 9

Day of Palsy	1	2	3	4	5	6	7	8	9	10	11	12	13	14	15	16	17	18	19	20	Not measurable
1st examination day			137 138	139	140			141					142							143 144 145	
End of degeneration phase							138			140			142		137					139	141 143 144 145
Deblocking begins																					

A glance at Table 3.1 is enough to show that in the majority of cases degeneration was completed by the 10th day. If the values could have been more closely plotted, an even higher proportion of cases would have fallen into this zone. This is because the end point was taken as the day on which the last examination showed no further decline in compound action potential amplitude (the exceptions will be discussed later). But in many cases an interval of several days occurred between this day and the previous measurement. The graph for case 71 shows, for example, that the 11th day of palsy is given for the degeneration end point. The measurement previous to this took place on the 6th day. So there were 5 days between the two measurements, and it seems not unreasonable to assume that if daily examinations had been carried out the point where there was no further decline in amplitude could have been located between the 8th and 9th days.

Table 3.1 shows that in 81, or 64.8%, of the cases evaluated in regard to this point, the degeneration phase had ended at the latest by the 10th day, and in 100 patients (or 80%) by the 11th day. Of the other 25 cases in which the degeneration phase had not ended by the 11th day, 8 (or 6.4%) showed an increase of more than 5%, and in only 4 patients (3.2%) was the increase more than 10% (cases 73, 84, 94, and 98).

What conclusions can be drawn from these findings for the actual events in the nerve? Fiber degeneration is not something that occurs in the nerve very suddenly. Even when a nerve is suddenly severed, it takes several days, depending on the distance of the particular section from the point of damage, before the "degeneration front" reaches the nerve ending. It is difficult to establish precisely the speed of advance of the degeneration front. In the ischemia model of Lundborg (1970) the n. tibialis degenerated over a period of 2–3 days in a section of 12–14 cm after a period of ischemia of 6 h. In the case of the facial nerve we can assume a section of 3.5–4 cm between the site of the lesion at the entry to the facial canal and the point of stimulation 0.5–1 cm distal from the stylomastoid foramen. This would indicate that when a nerve fiber starts to degenerate at the entry to the facial canal the "degeneration front" would arrive 1 or 2 days later at the point of stimulation behind the angle of the jaw ceases to react. If a sudden and complete ischemia occurred at the canal entry, the impulse conduction for voluntary innervation would be completely blocked within 30 min at most. Degeneration would start about 7 h later, and in 1 day, or 2 at the maximum, the stimulus point of the facial nerve at the stylomastoid foramen would no longer respond. However, we did not see a single case of such an apoplectic form of the degeneration phase. The earliest termination point for completed degeneration was in the case of idiopathic facial palsy by the 7th day of palsy (case 138), and also on the 7th day for herpes oticus (case Z12 and Z15). It should be noted, however, that in both the herpes cases the first examination occurred on the 7th day, so the possibility that the degeneration phase had ended earlier cannot be excluded.

If we work on the assumption that 1 or 2 days elapse before a nerve that has begun to degenerate at the facial canal entry ceases to react at the point of stimulation, it is logical to conclude that if the degeneration phase had been completed in 80% of patients by the 11th day of palsy, the events leading to degeneration at the canal entry had already terminated by the 9th or 10th day. If we include in these calculations the other 17 patients who showed no more than a further 5% degeneration by the 11th day, we can safely say that by the 10th day of palsy the degeneration phase had ended in 93% of patients.

Table 3.1. Idiopathic facial palsy (Group 1–9)

End of degeneration phase

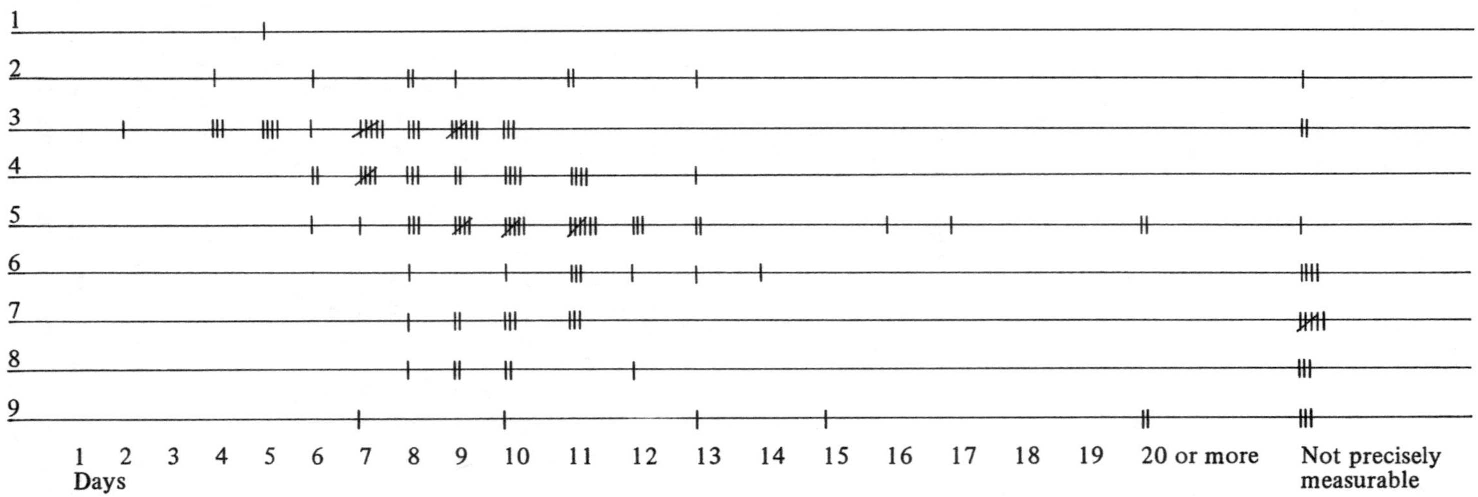

Of the remaining eight patients, four showed a further degeneration of up to 10% (cases 95, 106, 121, and 134). The graphs indicate that in these four cases 90% or more of the final degree of degeneration had been reached by the 11th day.

Of the other 4 patients (cases 73, 84, 94, and 98) only case 84 appears out of step. Here the degree of degeneration rose from 32% on the 11th day of palsy to 82% on the 28th day. A study of the graph shows that here there was a diphasic history: After the degeneration process had halted on the 7th day of palsy, it began again between the 11th and 15th days. In view of this phenomenon we might ask ourselves whether this was not a case of facial palsy of different pathogenesis, or else we have to assume that idiopathic facial palsy can at times depart from the norm and show a graph with two apexes.

In considering the graphs of cases 128, 129, and 130 (and in fact others), a slight decline in amplitude of the compound action potential of a few percent is noticeable after the 10th day of palsy. At the same time a sharp rise in latency can be observed, and this is particularly marked in case 129. A prolongation in the latency period indicates a slowing of the speed of conduction. So where in case 129 the latency triples there is a corresponding reduction of speed of conduction to one-third of the normal, that is, about 12 to 13 m/sec. Slowing of the impulse conduction does not affect all the fibers uniformly–it is more marked in some than in others. Since the latency data refer to the fibers where speed of conduction was highest, we have to take into account in the above example that in part of the fibers the conduction speed was still well under 12 m/sec. We must conclude that the result is a much increased dispersion of the compound action potential, which can lead to very strong polyphase. The increased scatter of compound action potential means not only that it lasts longer, but also that there is a decrease in amplitude. This decrease is not due to degeneration *but to desynchronization of* the discharges of *motor units.* We cannot therefore continue to regard the late phase of amplitude reduction of the compound action potential as being related to degeneration, particularly when it developes a much flatter gradient than that of the preceding very rapid phase of amplitude reduction. This is another reason not to accord a special classification to cases with a late phase of slight amplitude reduction.

In regard, therefore, to the evolution of the degeneration phase of idiopathic facial palsy it is possible to formulate the following principle:

In idiopathic facial palsy the degeneration of nerve fibers and the accompanying acute phase of nerve lesion are complete by the 10th day of palsy at the latest. Case 84 is an extreme case, or can simply be regarded as not belonging to the group at all, and is excluded. If it were not possible to exclude such cases, it would simply not be feasible to attempt to establish any rule or principle in biology.

A major advantage of the methods described in this work, and which represents considerable progress, is that it is possible not only to give details of the degree of nerve fiber degeneration, but also to go even beyond that and ascertain at what point the degeneration process ends. The two main aspects of the acute phase of nerve lesion, rapidity (velocity) and regularity, have not previously been brought out in the literature. This new insight, which rests on very solid evidence, has consequences for therapy which will be discussed later.

At this point another attempt should be made to identify more concretely the events at the entry to the facial canal. When strangulation of the nerve begins, a growing number of fibers will be blocked, depending on the force and rapidity (velocity) of the process. If the strangulation is not severe, and soon recedes, the impulse conduction block is reversible. However, if the strangulation lasts for any length of time, conduction block will become irreversible in a growing number of fibers. They must then degenerate. But such degeneration does not necessarily set in immediately—a latent pariod of several days can intervene between the time-point at which the destiny of the fiber is settled and the actual point in time when degeneration is actually completed. Let us refer again to the animal experiment for illustration: in Lundborg's tests the nerve's ultimate fate was settled after 7 h of ischemia. It had to degenerate. However, it still responded to stimulus for 2 to 3 days after this point in time had been reached. In Lundborg's experiments, ischemia started abruptly and was total. We are not likely to encounter such extreme conditions in the majority of cases of idiopathic facial palsy. In addition, it is also possible that function can be sustained, given certain minimal conditions, beyond the point where ultimate degeneration of the fiber has become certain. But it is difficult to say precisely how long it is before the end of the degeneration phase is recognizable that the situation becomes irreparable.

In conclusion, it is worth pointing out that it is not possible to make any systematic grouping of cases in regard to the end of the degeneration phase on the evidence of Table 3.1. In other words, the phase of degeneration will run its course in a period of time that is not affected one way or the other by the number of fibers involved.

2. *Conduction Block and the Beginning of its Recovery*

Whereas it is not possible to distinguish in any systematic way between groups 1 to 9 regarding the end point of nerve fiber degeneration, a study of Table 3.2b shows that there is a steady shift to the right in regard to the beginning of recovery from block (of those fibers that have escaped from degeneration) with increasing degrees of degeneration. This is particularly noticeable in groups 7 and 8, in which, with only two exceptions, the point where axon block begins to recede begins after the 20th day. Group 9 is not taken into consideration regarding this aspect, since all fibers have degenerated.

In groups 1 and 2, where degeneration was up to 30%, the paralysis began to recede in most cases already before the 10th day of palsy. Equilibrium is reached in group 3 (30–50% degeneration)—in about half the cases recovery from block began before the 10th day of palsy, and after that date in the others. In groups 5 and 6 the shift to the right is very evident.

If we take the average time between the 1st day of palsy and the beginning of recovery from block, we get the following results for groups 1 to 8:

Table 3.2a. Average period of latency between onset of palsy and beginning of recovery from block

Group	Days	
1	9.3	
2	10.3	
3	12.2	
4	13.2	
5	14.9	
6	17.3	
7	19.6	
8	20	or more

Three observations can be made in regard to this table: (1) The day which is entered for the beginning of recovery from block is that on which it was observed for the first time. Since the period between examinations varied from 1 to 4 days, recovery of block began 1 to 2 days before the date indicated, in some cases. But since this error affects all the groups equally, the differences between the groups remain unchanged. (2) The difference between groups 7 and 8 is in reality greater than would emerge from the figures given. As the table ends with the 20th day, the differences after that date are not shown. (3) If the need is felt to determine the point where recovery from block begins with more precision, an EMG can be made. With a coaxial needle electrode it is possible to record the first activity of motor units after complete block by as much as 1–2 days before the clinical signs of recovery appear.

Table 3.2 shows that in fact the final degree of degeneration of the nerve is a function of the degree of illness. In other words, it reflects to some extent that the capacity for recovery of the blocked fibers decreases in direct relation to the extent of degeneration, and this could indicate the severity of axonal damage. When, as we have shown in the previous section, the nerve fiber degeneration has ended by the 10th day of palsy at the latest, it can be assumed that from that point in time onwards the factors that are causing the damage are no longer strong enough to induce the degenerative process to continue. A kind of status quo arises, in which there is no further degeneration of fibers, but there is still no conduction. This is of course no more than the appearance of a stationary period, a transitional stage the length of which is directly related to the degree of degeneration. In limited degeneration it is short, and in more extensive degeneration it is more prolonged.

For an explanation of the differences in length of this transitional stage, the two most important hypotheses are: (1) When the degree of degeneration is severe, the damage to the blocked axons is greater in consequence, and they will therefore be subject to much more strain right up to the point where the process begins to reverse itself than where the degree of degeneration is low. It would seem natural that an axon that has suffered more damage will need more time to recover. (2) The longer period of block where there is greater degeneration could also be due to the fact that the processes that lead to strangulation of the nerve take longer to lose their momentum in severe cases than in mild ones.

We can express the difference between these two hypotheses in the following manner: In the first case the factors responsible for the length of the transitional stage are intra-axonal, and in the second are extra-axonal.

In Lundborg's tests with acute ischemia conduction block took 1.5 min to recover after 2-h ischemia, 3.5 min after 4-h ischemia, and 8 min after 6-h ischemia. There was no recovery after 8-h ischemia, indicating that the fibers had already degenerated to the point of no return. These results would seem to show that the point of no return can be reached suddenly. So long as some margin of time remains before it supervenes, the blocked axon can recover quite rapidly, providing, of course, that the factor causing damage has ceased to operate.

Unfortunately, the Lundborg experiments with acute ischemia cannot be considered sufficiently comparable to provide all the answers to the questions that have been raised here. However, there is another avenue worth exploring, which will be discussed in the next section.

Table 3.2 b. Idiopathic facial palsy (Group 1–9)

Deblocking begins

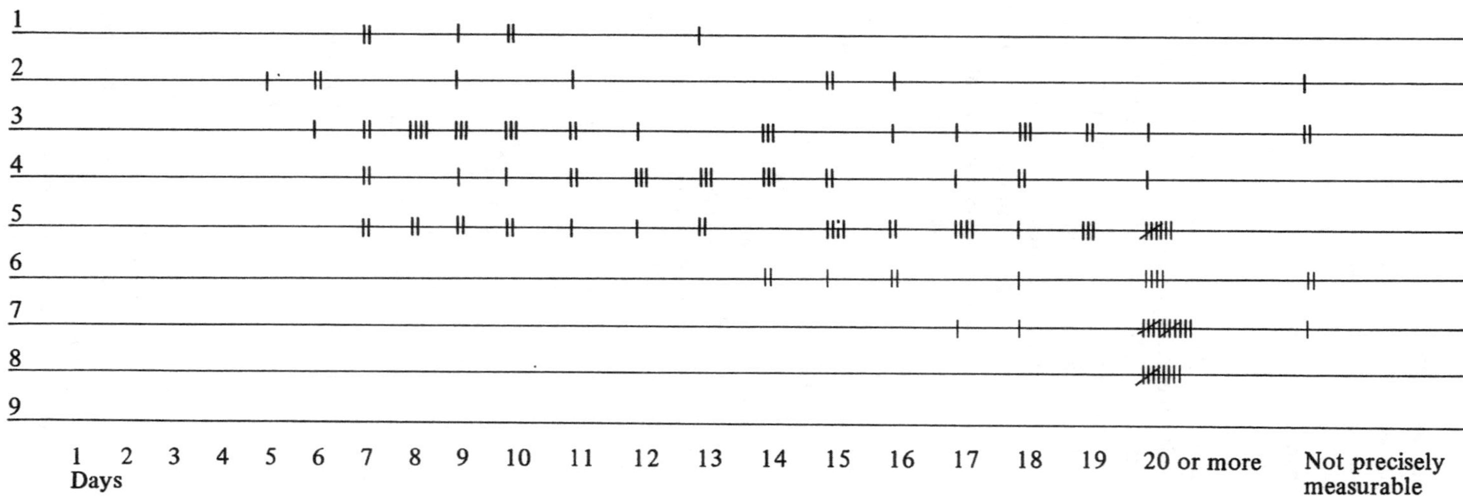

3. Latency

If the latencies of the individual cases are compared in the corresponding groups (see graph 9a–l), it is immediately clear that such periods increase progressively in length from one group to another. In most cases latency begins to lengthen on about the 5th day of palsy, and reaches a peak between the 15th and 40th days. In group 1 the latency remains constant throughout. In group 2 there is no sign of change in two of the selected cases, while the other three show a slight increase. However, the prolongation of latency is already more noticeable in groups 3 and 4. In group 5 (70–90% degeneration) for the first time all the latency curves show an increase, and in two cases this prolongation is considerable, rising to two-and-a-half to three times the initial value. There are similar patterns in group 6, but none of the more extreme values seen in group 5. This, obviously, is because a much smaller number of cases could be evaluated. In group 7 (95–98% degeneration) there is a further systematic increase in latency between the 4th and 8th day of palsy. The prolongation of latency is very strongly marked in group 8, reaching levels of between 12 and 16 ms, representing a four to fivefold increase of the initial value. Group 9 (100% degeneration) presents a special situation, in that in all cases the latency only reaches its full value when the degeneration of all fibers has been completed.

Another important finding emerges from a review of the latency graphs: a comparison of the graphs between individual groups brings out clearly the progressive increase in latency. At the same time there is a considerable amount of variation within a group There is no doubt that prolongation of the latency period correlates with the degree of severity of the nerve lesion, although this is only a statistical deduction and could not be used in individual cases as a clinical parameter.

We should now see what all these findings really represent in regard to the pathogenetic events in the facial nerve. Consider first the period of time between the impulse in the section of the nerve that lies behind the angle of the jaw and the emergence of compound action potential in the region of the perioral muscles. If this period shows an increase, it simply means that there is a decline in the speed of conduction of those facial nerve fibers that are distal to the block but still respond to stimulation. If the latency arises to three times the initial value, for example, then conduction speed falls to one-third, or from 35 to 40 m/s in normal cases to 12 or 13 m/s. If we bear in mind that on the one hand an increasing prolongation and polyphase of the compound action potential indicates increased dispersion, while on the other the latency indicates the velocity of conduction of the most rapid fibers, it is clear that deceleration of the speed of conduction will be more marked in some of the fibers.

If the facial nerve fibers show an increasing deceleration of conduction at a point 8–10 cm from the site of lesion at the entrance to the facial canal during the course of the disease, this indicates *that the local effect is also beginning to affect the whole length of the fibers.* An axon which conducts more slowly is diseased, and obviously the severity of disease is directly related to the deceleration involved. We know that the axons still capable of conduction do so more slowly at higher degrees of degeneration than at lower levels, and this indicates that they are more severely diseased. Investigation and analysis of variations in latency period provides the answer to the question of what causes the delay in recovery from block at the higher levels of degeneration. These variations must reflect the degree of severity of axonal disease which increases with the level of degeneration. Such axonal disease can last for a considerable period of time, as is shown by the fact that the prolongation of latency can often persist for months at a time. In some cases this prolongation can still be demonstrated after more than a year (e.g., cases 114, 117).

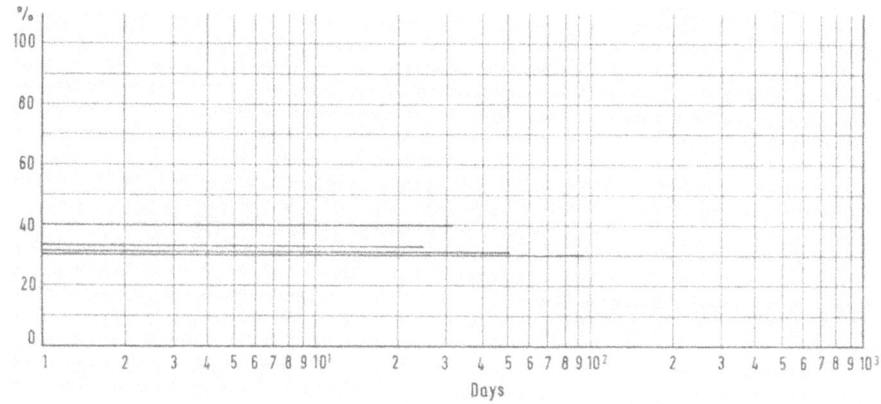

Fig. 8 a–i. Latencies in idiopathic facial palsy (group 1: 0–10% degeneration)

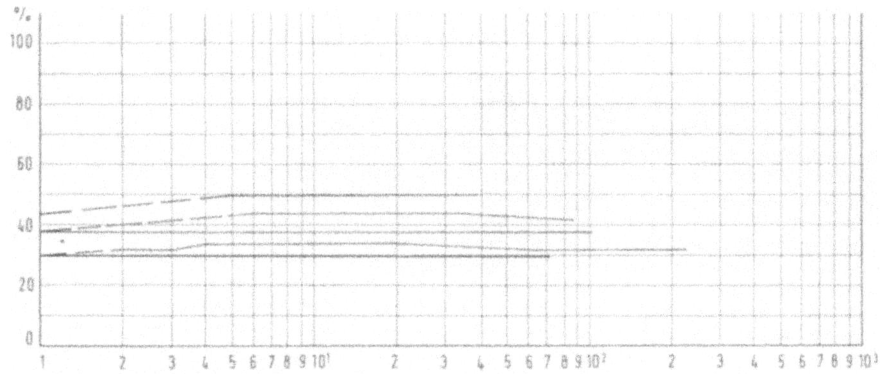

Fig. 8b (group 2: 10–30% degeneration)

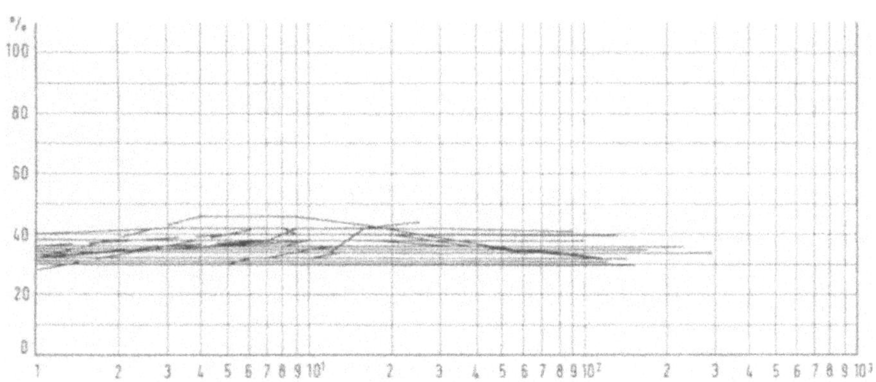

Fig. 8c (group 3: 30–50% degeneration)

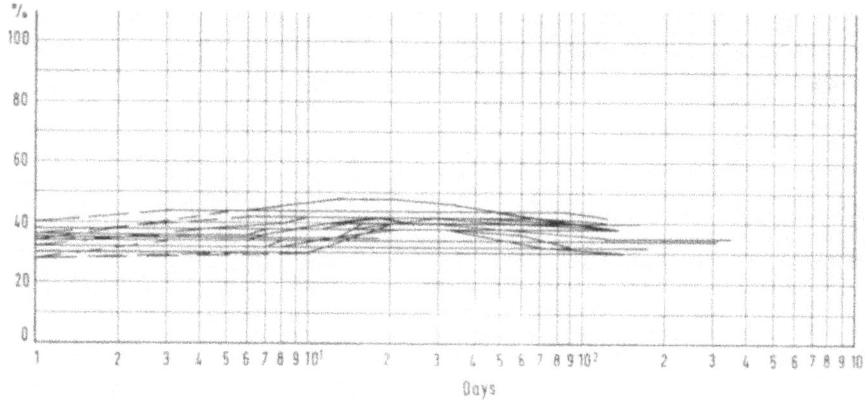

Fig. 8d (group 4: 50–70% degeneration)

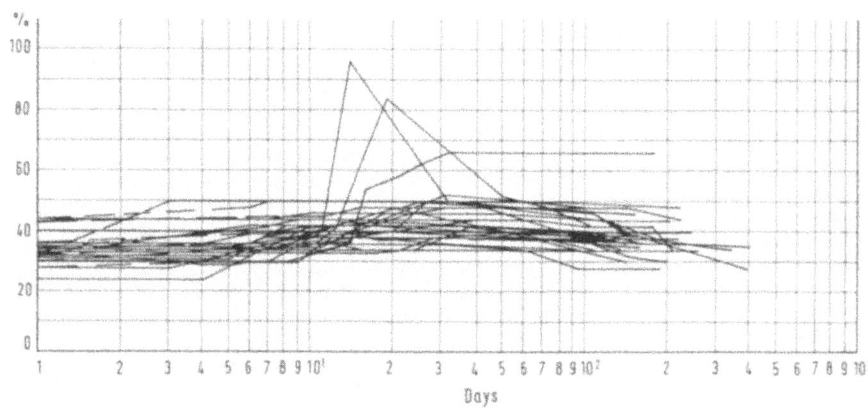

Fig. 8e (group 5: 70–90% degeneration)

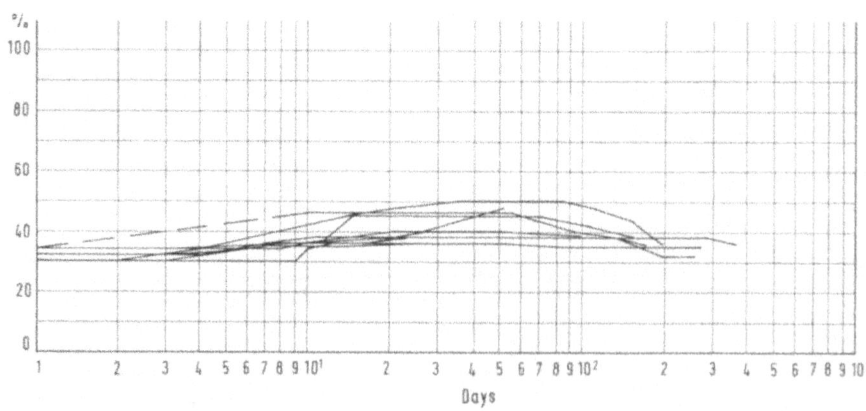

Fig. 8f (group 6: 90–95% degeneration)

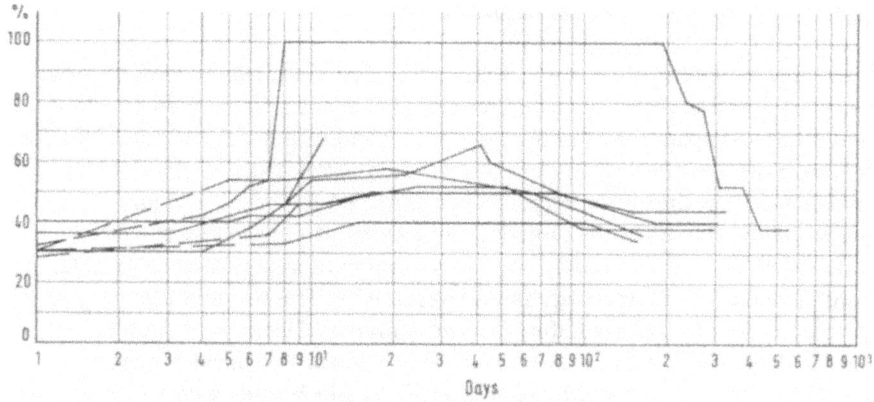

Fig. 8g (group 7: 95–98% degeneration)

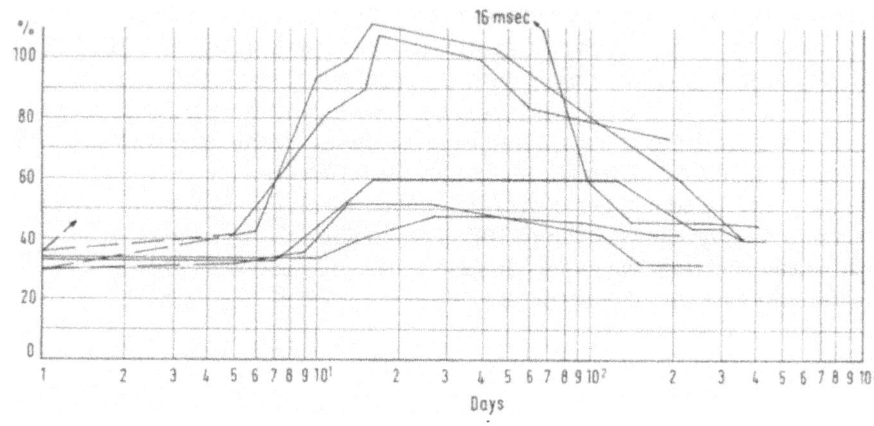

Fig. 8h (group 8: 98–99% degeneration)

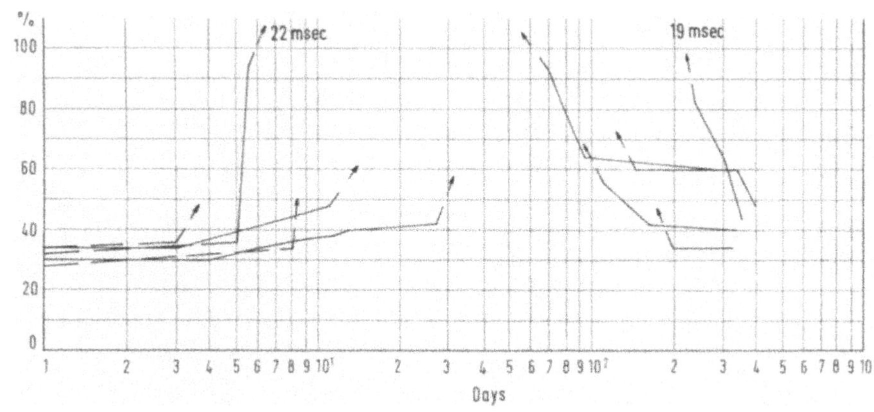

Fig. 8i (group 9: 100% degeneration)

4. Completion of Recovery from Conduction Block

In most cases the end-point of recovery from conduction block can be read off from the graph, since the (thick) "palsy curve" reaches a plateau and from then on evolves with a flatter line (compare for example cases 48, 59 and 69). In case 48 the beginning of recovery from block on the 18th day of palsy onset is clearly recognizable. The "palsy curve", or what in this connection might be better named the "recovery curve", then climbs quite steeply, that is, in the direction of recovery of function by the facial muscles. By the 40th day only a slight residuum of plasy of about 5% is detectable, or in other words there is a recovery reaching a level of 95%. This residuum takes markedly longer to recede than that between the 18th and 40th day. Clearly it is essential that a portion of the denervated facial muscles be reinnervated for this phase of recovery. *The improvement of facial innervation can as a rule be ascribed up to the 40th day of palsy onset rather to the recovery of conductance of blocked fibers than to regeneration of degenerated fibers.*

Axon block does not always recede at the same rate. Even within a single group there will be variations of from one to two weeks in length, and in certain cases much longer. It should also be kept in mind that after the 20th day of palsy onset the patient examinations could not in every case be carried out frequently enough to make it possible to fix the end-point of recovery from block with complete precision. An allowance for error of from 10 to 15 days has to be made. But since this applies to all groups, it is still possible to make a systematic analysis of the differences.

The end-points for complete recovery from block are set out by group in Table 3.3. Up to, and including, group 4 (i.e. up to 70% degeneration), there are no really noteworthy differences between the groups. In general, the process takes from 4 to 6 weeks, counting from the first day of palsy onset.

Table 3.3. End of deblocking

Case	Day of Palsy	20	30	40	50	60	70	80	not measurable
	1			x					
	2			x					
	3		x						
1	4			x					
	5		x						
	6							x	
	7	x							
	8		x						
	9								x
	10		x						
	11			x					
2	12			x					
	13								x
	14			x					
	15			x					
	16			x					
	17		x						
	18			x					
	19		x						
	20			x					
	21					x			
	22								x
	23			x					
	24								x
	25		x						
	26		x						
	27		x						
	28			x					
	29								x
3	30		x						
	31		x						
	32		x						
	33			x					
	34							x	
	35	x							
	36		x						
	37		x						
	38			x					
	39		x						
	40		x						
	41			x					
	42			x					
	43		x						
	44			x					
	45			x					
	46								x
	47			x					
	48			x					
	49						x		
	50			x					
4	51								x
	52								x
	53		x						
	54		x						
	55			x					
	56		x						
	57		x						
	58								x
	59		x						
	60		x						
	61								x
	62								x
	63			x					
	64		x						
	65								x
	66	x							
	67		x						
	68								x
	69		x						
	70								x
	71				x				
	72		x						
	73			x					
	74					x			
	75		x						
	76			x					
	77								x
	78			x					
	79		x						
	80							x	
	81		x						
	82								x
	83								x
5	84		x						
	85					x			
	86		x						
	87		x						
	88								x
	89		x						
	90			x					
	91								x
	92					x			
	93								x
	94								x
	95					x			
	96		x						

Table 3.3. End of deblocking (continued)

Case	Day of Palsy	20	30	40	50	60	70	80	not measurable
	97								x
	98								
	99		x						
	100			x					
	101		x						
	102								x
	103			x					
	104					x			
6	105								x
	106			x					
	107				x				
	108							x	
	109				x				
	110			x					
	111								x
	112								x
	113		x·						
	114		x						
	115								x
	116								x
	117								x
	118				x				
	119		x						
7	120				x				
	121					x			
	122								x
	123								x
	124							x	
	125								x
	126				x				
	127								x
	128			x					
	129					x			
	130								x
	131								x
8	132				x				
	133						x		
	134								x
	135								x
	136						x		

The acute phase of illness can be considered to last 10 days, during which the degeneration of facial nerve fibers takes place and there is no possibility of recovery of conductance by the blocked fibers except for slight degrees of degeneration. The actual period of recovery, at the end of which the greater part of the blocked fibers are again conducting, is accordingly reduced to between 2 and 4 weeks.

From group 5 (70–90% degeneration) onwards, the spread of the recovery period is, as Table 3.3 demonstrates, markedly greater. However, even in this group the recovery of conductance can be completed in a relatively short time. In some cases, however (notably cases 80, 108, and 124), it can still drag on for some time—up to 80 days. This also applies, incidentally, for certain cases in groups 1 to 4 (case 6, 34). Perhaps in these cases a residual edema of the facial nerve remains at the entrance to the canal which prevents some—although not the greater part—of the blocked fibers from recovering. It will be recalled that in other nerves, e.g., in compression paralysis of the radial or peroneal nerve, conduction block can last up to 3 months.

On the whole, however, it must be said that the differences between groups for the parameter of completion of recovery from block is very slight, and no real pattern can be discerned. This is clearly due to the fact that completion of recovery from block correlates with the parameter of "end of degeneration phase", which, as we have seen already (see pp. 66–70), shows no group-specific characteristics. Once degeneration has been completed, recovery from block in the case of a high level of degeneration starts somewhat later (see pp. 71–73). However this initial delay is again partly compensated for during the further evolution of this phase.

Once recovery from block is complete, the "palsy curve" or "recovery curve" (*medium*) is always above the degeneration curve (*thick*), i.e., the residual degree of palsy is in all cases less significant than the degeneration curve would lead one to expect in theory.

The clinically observable degree of recovery is always better than the degeneration curve would indicate, and both curves reach their widest point of separation at the end of the recovery from block. This important principle, which has emerged for the first time as a result of the investigatory techniques and general standpoint under discussion here, will be further considered later (pp. 83–89).

5. *Degree of Nerve Regeneration*

The regenerative processes begin directly from the nerve fiber degeneration phase. Two important proliferative processes must be distinguished. One originates at the proximal end of the axon, the other in the Schwann cells of the degenerated section of the nerve fiber distal to the point of lesion. The proliferating Schwann cells form into ribbons, sometimes known as Büngner's ribbons, which act as guide channels for the axonal proliferative process (Sunderland, 1968; Kreutzberg, in Miehlke, 1973).

The speed of regeneration of a nerve fiber, and ultimately of the whole nerve, depends, as has been pointed out elsewhere, very much on the condition of the nerve connective tissue. If the mesenchymal nerve fiber sheaths have remained intact (axonotmesis), the regeneration process is rapid, corresponding to the speed of axoplasma flow of 1–3 mm per day (Gutmann, 1955). In particularly favorable conditions the rate can increase to as much as 5 mm per day. When the regenerating nerve fibers reach the area of neuromuscular junction, the motor end-plate, which is usually also affected, has to be reconstructed. If we are using only physiologic and morphologic criteria, it is true to say that regeneration is successful when the first impulses arriving at the nerve fiber terminal release sufficient ACh to depolarize the reconstructed end-plate to the critical level when a propagated depolarization of the muscle fiber membrane is triggered.

But the motor units system is not restored to function quite so quickly. The newly regenerated fibers still conduct impulses with less speed, and the neuromuscular junction is not yet capable of transmitting the higher discharge rates, and tires quickly. It takes weeks before the motor units really begin to function efficiently.

A question that is worth raising now is whether we can establish the earliest point at which regeneration can be detected, using the methods described in this work. If we take as a basis a length of 30 mm for the facial canal, and 80–90 mm from the stylomastoid foramen to the area of the perioral muscles, then the regenerating nerve fibers must attain a length of about 120 mm before their activity can be picked up either by electromyography or by electroneurography.

Assuming an average regeneration rate of 1 mm per day we could expect to see the first signs of regeneration in 120 days, since we must allow for a 10-day degeneration phase in 130 days following onset of palsy. If a regeneration rate of 3 mm per day is assumed, regeneration would be completed after 50 days, and in exceptional cases where the rate was even faster we could expect to record signs of regeneration within 5 weeks after the 1st day of palsy. It must be kept in mind, of course, that only a portion of the fibers will regenerate so quickly. But what matters is that there should as a general rule be an increase in amplitude of the compound action potential in the 6th week of palsy.

A review of the history tables shows that in fact in some cases there is an increase in amplitude between the 30th and 50th days. However, we are not concerned here so much with these "record breakers", as with systematic differentiation between the groups. For the latter purpose, the degrees of regeneration in Table 3.4 can be classified according to periods of 60–80 days, 90–120 days, 180–220 days, and 300 and 400 days. In each individual case we have to determine by what percentage the amplitude curve rose again from its lowest point to the point of comparison, and then calculate the average of the amplitude increases for each group.

Table 3.4 shows a rise in the regeneration degree of 17–21% between groups 1 and 2 over the 60–80 day period. But it would be erroneous to conclude that the regeneration rate was more rapid in group 2. The difference is more apparent than real, and arises because group 2 (up to 30% degeneration) has a higher degree of degeneration, and can thus produce a greater "amount" of regeneration than group 1. The same applies in regard to the increase of the degree of regeneration in the period 90–120 days. The apparent regeneration rises from group 1 (21%) to group 3 (37%) but again only because group 3 (up to 50% degeneration) can produce a greater amount of regeneration in this period than group 1 or group 2.

Table 3.4. Degree of regeneration in idiopathic facial palsy

Day of palsy	60–80	90–120	180–220	300	400	500
Group: 1						
2	17%	21%				
3	22%	30%				
4	18.4%	37%				
5	18.2%	34.2%	52.6%			
6	10.5%	15.8%	26%	36.5%		
7		16.0%	26%	32%	37%	
8		4.2%	14.7%	34%		
9		2.0%	11%	19.3%		

The fall-off in degree of regeneration shown in Table 3.4 between group 5 (up to 90% degeneration) and group 6 (up to 95% degeneration) in the time period 60–80 days must, on the other hand, be accepted as accurately reflecting the situation. The rate of regeneration evolves progressively more slowly in groups 6 to 8 (90–99% degeneration). This emerges even more clearly when a comparison is made of the time periods 90–120 and 180–220 days. The degree of regeneration falls off sharply between group 5 and 6. But in this regard no difference can be observed between group 6 (90–95% degeneration) and group 7 (96–97% degeneration). On the other hand, group 8 (98–99% degeneration) shows another sharp fall-off of the degree of regeneration compared to group 7. In group 9 the amount of regeneration is again halved. By 200 days group 9 still has not reached the degree of regeneration that was achieved in group 7 by the 100th day. In fact, group 9 does not reach this level until the 300th day.

There can be no doubt that the poor showing by groups 8 and 9 must be attributed to the much greater damage to nerve connective tissue at the site of strangulation.

6. *Degree of Functional Recovery*

This heading covers the whole functional picture, i.e., the clinical evaluation of the degree to which palsy recedes. As has been already demonstrated in Section 3.3.0, the investigator himself introduces an unavoidably subjective element into the evaluation process. As the basis for such an estimation the investigator has to make a judgement concerning the extent to which there is an innervation-linked asymmetry of the most mimetic movements (showing the teeth, pursing the lips to whistle, closing the eyes, wrinkling the forehead), as well as the ability to close one eye independently of the other. This latter test can continue to reveal a residuum of palsy, even when mimetic symmetry has already been fully restored. According to the degree of disability, this test can be used to estimate a residuum of palsy of 5–10%, indicating a degree of functional recovery of 90–95%. Another test–and sometimes the only one–that can be used to detect the residuum of a facial palsy is the eyelash sign (signe de cils). At maximal eyelid closure the eyelashes on the affected side do not meet as completely as on the other. If this were the only sign of a residuum, it would be rated at 5% (a 95% degree of functional recovery).

A brief reference has already been made in the section on completion of recovery from conduction block to the fact that the "palsy curve", or "recovery curve" will in most cases tend to be congruent with the degeneration curve at the end of the recovery phase (cf., for example cases 48, 59, and 69). When all fibers that have been blocked have recovered their conduction capacity, purely clinical observation would indicate a much lower degree of damage to the nerves than would be shown de facto from the degeneration curve. In case 48, for example, a clinical estimation on the 40th day of palsy indicated a residuum of 5%, or an almost complete functional recovery, while the degeneration curve showed a degree of degeneration of fully 50%. The difference was even more marked in case 69 and others.

This discrepancy between the functional recovery curve and the degeneration curve refers only to observable facial function, i.e., with a palsy degree of 0, or a recovery degree of 100, no difference between one side of the face and the other can be detected even in vigorous grimacing. However, when the strength of individual muscles of the face is measured, it can be seen to be fully in proportion to the degree of innervation as it can be judged from the amplitude or degeneration curve. Measurement of the strength of facial muscles in this way can be carried out fairly easily with the aid of a spring balance. The movable arm of the balance is taped tightly to the muscle (e.g., to the frontal muscle or to the orbicular muscle of the eye). The balance is then loaded to the point where the strength of the maximally innervated facial muscle is overcome, and the corresponding value read off. If this is compared with the same muscle on the other side, it is easy to compute the difference in strength on the paretic side.

Degrees of degeneration of up to 50% of the facial nerve fibers are not clinically detectable providing that the remaining fibers maintain their conduction intact. This finding has important implications which will be discussed more fully later on.

The rate and extent of functional recovery for the individual groups can be seen from Table 3.5. Nonetheless it is useful at this stage to correlate the percentage with a qualitative scale in order to refine assessment of the clinical efficacity of functional recovery:

Degree of functional recovery %	Clinical evaluation
100	Very good
90–100	Good
80– 90	Satisfactory
70– 80	Fair
50– 70	Unsatisfactory
30– 50	Poor
under 30	Very poor.

In group 1 the recovery from paralysis was completed between the 20th and 40th days after onset of palsy (inclusive of day of onset) with the exception of case 6, where the reversal of axon block was unduly protracted.

In all nine patients in group 2 the evolution could be followed up to complete recovery from paralysis. In four cases it was complete by up to the 40th day, and in the other five between the 40th and 80th days.

The spread was much greater in group 3 (30–50% degeneration). Of the 27 measurable cases 11 showed recovery from palsy up to the 40th day, while the others fell into a period extending from the 40th to the 120th day.

Of the 17 measurable cases in group 4 only one had complete functional recovery by the 40th day. In the others it took from 40 to 160 days. Nevertheless, recovery was very good in all the cases in this group.

In group 5 (70–90% degeneration) this was not always the case, however. Most of the 32 patients needed over 100 days for complete recovery from palsy. In 21 patients full clinical recovery of function was reached by up to the 200th day. In those cases where there was still some residual palsy by the 200th day, it was so slight that recovery of function could be recorded either as good or at least satisfactory. In all probability a longer period of observation would have shown a good, or even very good final result for all patients.

In group 6 (90–95% degeneration) some cases could first of all be observed with a degree of recovery from palsy that could not be placed higher than fair, and others that were unsatisfactory. Nevertheless a complete recovery from palsy was reached in 5 of the 11 patients, even though in some the process took up to 300 days.

The functional end result remained clearly unsatisfactory in case 108. Both at the 200th and again at the 300th day there remained a 50% paralysis in this 34-year-old patient, and further improvement can no longer be expected. Yet such a poor end result comes as a surprise when the amplitude curve is studied on this patient's history. The graph alone would indicate that a considerable recovery of function could be

Table 3.5. Degree of restitution in facial palsy

Day of palsy		30	40	50	60	70	80	90	100	120	140	160	180	200	300	400	500	600
	Case 7				100													
	8		100															
	9					100												
	10		100															
2	11		100															
	12		100															
	13						100											
	15			100														
	16									100								
	17		100															
	18						100											
	19	100																
	20		100															
	21				100													
	22			100														
	24				100													
	25	100																
	26			100														
	27		100															
3	28	100																
	29					100												
	30					100												
	31		100															
	32					100												
	33		100															
	34									100								
	35				100													
	36				100													
	37			100														
	38					100												
	39		100															
	40	100																
	41		100															
	42								100									
	43								100									
	44							100										
	45						100											

Table 3.5. Degree of restitution in facial palsy (continued)

Day of palsy		30	40	50	60	70	80	90	100	120	140	160	180	200	300	400	500	600
	47						100											
	48						100											
	49					100												
	50						100											
	52									95								
	53								100									
	54				100													
	55									100								
4	56											100						
	57							100										
	58								100									
	59				100													
	60						100											
	61			100														
	62				100													
	63		100															
	64					100												
	66				100													
	67											80						
	68										100							
	69										100							
	70											85						
	71			100														
	72								100									
	73												100					
	74													100				
	75						100											
	76												100					
	77													100				
	78													100				
	79					100												
	80													85			90	
	81											100						
	83													100				
5	84											100						
	85												100					

Table 3.5. Degree of restitution in facial palsy (continued)

Day of palsy		30	40	50	60	70	80	90	100	120	140	160	180	200	300	400	500	600
	86									100								
	87									70								
	89													80				
	90									100								
	91								100									
	92													80				
	93								100									
	94											95						
	95													95				
	96													100				
	97								95									
	98												100					
	99				100													
	100													100				
	101													100				
	103													100				
	104													90	95			
	105								50									
6	106													95				
	107										100							
	108													50	50			
	109										100							
	110													95	100			
	111													60				
	112													95				
	113													10	20			
	114										50			20	20			
	117													70	80	80		
	118								70			80						
	119													85	90	90		
7	120											50		70	90			
	121											85		90		100		
	122											100						
	123													100				
	124													70	80			

Table 3.5. Degree of restitution in facial palsy (continued)

Day of palsy		30	40	50	60	70	80	90	100	120	140	160	180	200	300	400	500	600
	125										100							
	126														90			
	127											50			60			
	128													35				
	129													50				
	130													100				
	131													20		60		
8	132													80	85			
	133													30	40	40		
	134													5	30			
	135														50			
	136													95				
	137														25			
	138													20	30	30		
	139													30	30	45		
9	140													50	80			
	141													10	20			
	142													40	50			
	143													95	95			
	144													20	50			70
	145																	

expected, and particularly that there would be an amelioration between the 200th and 300th days, because during this period the degree of degeneration fell from 77% to 57%. At the latter level other patients usually show a recovery from palsy that can at least be described as good. But the apparent contradiction is resolved by the observation that this patient showed marked associated movement (synkinesis) as early as the 200th day. Such synkinesis is, as has been pointed out by other writers, the result of misdirection of the regenerating axon. These errors arise when nerve connective tissue, and above all the endoneural tubes, are more badly damaged. Other cases in this group also showed synkinesis (for example cases 110 and 112), but it was so slight that functional recovery was not materially affected.

Three points emerge from an analysis of group 6: (1) Where the degree of degeneration is from 90–95% there is so much damage to the connective tissue in some patients that the regenerating axons cannot find the connection to the correct muscles, and misdirection occurs. (2) If such misdirection occurs in many fibers they are more likely to be the cause of a poor functional end result than any deficiency in the number of regenerating axons. (3) If synkinesis also occurs to any important degree, electroneurography can no longer be relied upon to indicate the quality of regeneration. The amplitude shows only the number of excitable motor units or muscle fibers, but will not give any information as to whether they are being supplied by the correct nerve fibers.

In group 7 (95–98% degeneration) there was an evolution lasting at the very least more than 300 days, and often much longer, in 12 of the 15 patients. Three of these showed very good recovery of function. In one the result was unsatisfactory, and in another it was poor. Several patients in this group also showed synkinesis, but none so marked as case 108 in group 6. In the patient with the poorest result (case 113) this could be ascribed, not to misdirection, but to unsufficient regeneration. At 300 days, the compound action potential in this 70-year-old man indicated a degree of degeneration of 82%, and there was only 15% regeneration.

Generally speaking, group 7 showed no worsening of the trends compared with group 6. However, the picture is quite different in the following groups.

Of the seven patients in group 8 (98–99% degeneration) who could be followed for 300 days or longer, only one showed very good recovery of function, and one other showed good recovery. In another patient it was satisfactory. In two patients recovery of function was unsatisfactory and in two others poor.

The retreat of palsy ranged from unsatisfactory to poor in more than half the patients. Those patients with the most unfavourable evolution usually had mor or less marked associated movement and facial contracture.

Evolution could be followed for a period of from more than 300 up to 500 days in eight patients in group 9 (complete degeneration). One of the eight showed a good recovery, another a satisfactory recovery, and the third was fair. In the other five the result was poor or very poor. All the patients with a poor result had associated movement and facial contracture of marked extent. These cases, in which an important contributory factor to the poor recovery from palsy was associated movement, i.e., misdirection of regenerating axons, could be easily identified on the graphs by the narrowing of the distance between the amplitude and palsy curves. In the case of very marked misdirection the palsy curve can fall below the amplitude curve (case 141), i.e., the degree of regeneration of the nerve fibers is markedly better than the degree of functional recovery from the palsy. If it were not for these misdirections, it seems likely that a number of patients with a poor end result would have had a satisfactory recovery of function.

The correlation between regeneration of the nerve fibers and recovery of mimetic function leads to the following conclusions:

1. Up to a degree of degeneration of 50% a very good recovery of function is achieved in every case, and this takes no more than 6 to 7 weeks in the majority of cases.

2. Up to a degree of degeneration of 90% a very good recovery of function is nearly always achieved, even though in a small number of cases a slight residual palsy remains—so slight that it is seldom noticeable to the layman. But by comparison with patients with a degree of degeneration of under 50%, the period of recovery of function in this group is considerably longer, and may be as much as threefold.

3. Up to a degree of degeneration of 90–98% the majority of patients achieve a satisfactory mimetic function, and in some cases recovery is in fact very good. Only in a small number of cases is the end result poor, and then often in association with misdirection of regenerated axons. The latter phenomenon only becomes noticeable at this degree of degeneration.

4. At 98–100% degeneration recovery of function is in most cases in a range from unsatisfactory to poor. Exceptions do occur, however, and some patients with this degree of degeneration achieve good and even very good recovery of function.

7. Age

Two lines of investigation can be pursued in regard to the age factor in idiopathic facial palsy:

1. Is there a correlation between severity (degree of degeneration) and age?
2. Can a correlation be established between age and degree and rate of regeneration?

The average age of the 145 patients with idiopathic facial palsy was 34. The youngest was 10, and the eldest 76. No significant correlation emerges when the average age of the individual groups is studied in relation to degree of degeneration, as the following table makes clear:

Table 3.6

Group	Average age	Age range
1	32.0	14–45
2	42.3	19–70
3	31.8	12–69
4	44.2	13–76
5	45.4	14–69
6	42.3	16–71
7	34.6	12–69
8	41.1	10–73
9	40.8	19–72

Thus group 1, with the lowest degree of degeneration, shows also one of the lowest age averages, while on the other hand the age average of group 5 (70–90% degeneration) at 45.4 is higher than in group 9 where, with total degeneration, the age average is 40.8.

In order to explore further the questions raised at the opening of this section, the age group 10–20 years was compared with the 60–70 years group.

Both groups, fortuitously, had 14 patients. A comparison of their histories in one graph (Fig. 11) does not produce any clear picture. Next we can calculate the average degree of degeneration for each age group on the 20th, 70th, and 100th days of palsy. The results are as set out in the following table:

Table 3.7

Day of palsy	20		70		100	
Age group	[a)] 1	2	1	2	1	2
	5	24	0	0	0	0
	29	31	0	22	0	15
	31	52	12	28	0	18
	39	62	18	36	0	23
	45	69	20	42	5	33
	48	70	36	48	15	44
	48	72	40	57	29	54
	55	75	52	67	46	70
	80	79	62	72	55	72
	82	81	69	78	61	77
	94	92	76	83	69	82
	95	93	77	85	70	95
	96	97	94	97	92	96
	99	99	96	99	95	97
Average degree of degeneration	60.4	71.1	46.5	58.1	38.3	55.1
% in favor of age group 1	15		20		31	

[a)] 1. 10–20 years
2. 60–70 years

At the 20th day of palsy the difference between the degrees of degeneration stands at 10.6% in favor of the 10–20 age group. If the degree of degeneration of the 60–70 age group = 100, the 10–20 age group shows a 15% lower degeneration. The divergence is even more marked at the 70th day of palsy with a figure of 20%, and by the 100th day it reaches 31%. These figures clearly demonstrate that average maximal degree of degeneration in the 10–20 age group is lower than in the 60–70 age group. The difference is even more marked in regard to regeneration, which develops much more quickly in the first group than in the second.

When average age of patients is used as a base for comparison of the best degrees of recovery of function with the worst, it is even more striking to note the facial nerve's much grater capability to regenerate in the younger patients. Groups 8 and 9, where the degree of degeneration is highest, are the most suitable choice for such a comparison. We find six patients with good or very good recovery of function on the one side, and seven with poor or very poor recovery on the other. The average age of the first group is 27.8 years, and the average age for the second is 53.0 years.

3.4.3. Herpes Oticus (Groups 1 and 2)

For reasons of space, the clinical symptoms will be described only very briefly.

Of the 21 cases there were 6 who had clear signs of damage to the vestibularis fibers, and another 6 with symptoms of a lesion of the vestibularis combined with damage to the cochlearis. Altogether, therefore, a total of 12 of the 21 patients had clear signs of a vestibularis lesion, which both clinically and in tests with apparatus manifested itself as both spontaneous and position nystagmus as well as fixation nystagmus. The clinical equivalent was a marked rotational or staggering vertigo, which in some cases lasted for several months. But absence of excitability in the labyrinth did not develop in any patient.

In some of the patients there was accompanying hearing difficulty, due to a disturbance of sound conduction. Damage to the cochlearis was not assumed until the hearing difficulty could be shown on the audiogram. The usual range was from –20 dB to –80 dB. The hearing difficulty retreated over a period of weeks or months.

No patient had cochlearis damage without an acompanying lesion of the vestibularis.

Group 1 (50–95% degeneration)
Cases Z1–Z7
Sex: 4 male, 3 female
Localization: 2 right, 5 left
Average age: 40.4 (22–57 years)

Z1: H. S., male, 51 years. On 10/10/73 pains and herpes eruptions, left side head, face, neck, auricle, and tympanic membrane. 10/18/73 facial palsy, left side. 10/25/73 vestibularis symptoms.

Z2: D. M., female, 53 years. On 5/1/73 pains in the ears. 5/9/73 swelling and herpes eruptions. Left auricle, vertigo. 5/11/73 facial palsy left side.

Z3: V. R., male, 42 years. On 8/1/72 pains in left ear. 8/4/72 facial palsy, left side. 8/6/72 swelling and herpes vesicles, left auricle. 8/10/72 vestibularis symptoms and hearing difficulty. Transtemporal decompression.

Z4: O. L., female, 57 years. On 10/20/71 buzzing in left ear. 10/23/71 pains in left ear. 10/24/71 lacrimation, burning, left eye. 10/26/71 facial palsy, left, marked vertigo. 10/28/71 hearing difficulty, left. 10/29/71 transtemporal decompression.

Z5: H. G., female, 29 years. On 10/28/72 herpes blisters, mouth, nose, palatine arch left. 11/4/72 facial palsy, left. 11/8/72 vertigo, spontaneous nystagmus. 11/13/72 hearing difficulty.

Z6: A. Z. male, 22 years. 11/11/73 herpes blisters, right side of neck and face. 11/14/73 rotational vertigo, vomiting, spontaneous nystagmus. Facial palsy, right. Hearing difficulty.

Z7: B. L., male, 29 years. 11/20/73 pains, right ear. 11/24/73 rotational vertigo, tendency to fall to right. 11/26/73 facial palsy, right. Hearing difficulty, spontaneous nystagmus, position nystagmus, vertigo.

Group 2 (95–100% degeneration)
Cases Z8–Z21
Sex: 7 male, 7 female
Localization: 6 right, 8 left
Average age: 46.9 years (19–76 years)

Z8: M. H., male, 55 years. 12/15/72 herpes eruptions, left side, neck, face, tympanic membrane. 12/21/72 facial palsy, left, hearing difficulty at high pitch, spontaneous and position nystagmus, vertigo. 12/22/72 transtemporal decompression (2nd day of palsy). By 4th day of palsy degeneration degree of 98%. No further deterioration. First signs of recovery of function and regeneration about 11th day. Satisfactory recovery up to 250th day, so that the patient could return to his occupation as clarinet player in an orchestra.

Z9: A. L., female, 55 years. 3/20/73 herpes eruption, left side neck (C1 and C2). 3/28/73 facial palsy, left.

Z10: E. P., female, 44 years. 4/16/71 pains, left ear. 4/19/71 tinnitus. 4/25/71 facial palsy left, rotational vertigo, hearing difficulty, spontaneous nystagmus. 5/2/71 (8th day of palsy) transtemporal decompression.

Z11: R. L., female, 47 years. 12/5/73 pains, left ear. 12/7/73 herpes eruption right, tympanum, facial palsy, right.

Z12: U. W. male, 28 years. 5/8/74 pains, left ear. 5/10/74 herpes eruption and swelling, left tympanum, facial palsy, left. 5/17/74 (8th day of palsy) transtemporal decompression.

Z13: R. B., male 56 years, 3/24/73 herpes eruption, right ear. 3/26/73 vertigo, vomitting. 4/11/73 facial palsy right. 4/6/73 spontaneous nystagmus.

Z14: J. H., female, 21 years. 3/1/73 pains, left ear. 3/2/73 facial palsy, left. 3/6/73 herpes eruption and swelling, left tympanum. 3/8/73 rotational vertigo to right, unsteady gait, loss of hearing, spontaneous nystagmus. 3/10/73 (8th day of palsy) transemporal decompression–history shows a moderately satisfactory regeneration of nerve fibers, but poor recovery of function following severe associated movement.

Z15: E. P., female, 65 years. 11/15/72 facial palsy left. 11/6/72 vertigo, vomiting, spontaneous nystagmus. Hearing difficulty.

Z 16: G. H. female, 61 years. 3/23/73 facial palsy left. 3/25/73 pains, left ear. 3/28/73 herpes eruption, left tympanum, internal auditory meatus. 3/31/73 (9th day of palsy) transtemporal decompression. For external reasons the case could not be followed up.

Z17: B. Z., male, 31 years. 3/13/74 herpes eruption, thoracic region, Th8, right. On same day facial palsy, right, ear pains. 3/21/74 (9th day of palsy) transtemporal decompression.

Z18: E. R., male, 38 years. 6/11/73 ear pains. 6/4/73 facial palsy, right. 6/6/73 Herpes eruption and swelling, right tympanum, spontaneous nystagmus.

Z19: B. L., male, 19 years. 1/28/71 facial palsy, right. 2/4/71 herpes eruption and swelling, right tympanum. 2/24/71 (28th day of palsy) transtemporal decompression. Postoperative follow-up was for external reasons only possible on the 700th and 1000th days.

Z20: F. M. female, 61 years. 3/7/73 ear pains, herpes eruption and swelling, right tympanum. 3/9/73 facial palsy, right.

Z21: C. F., male 76 years. 6/19/73 ear pains, herpes eruption, left tympanum. Facial palsy, left. Hearing difficulty on both sides and no response to stimulus in either labyrinth (probably due to age).

3.4.4. Principles of Disease Evolution in Facial Palsy Associated with Herpes Oticus

1. End of degeneration. Of the seven cases in group Z1 (50–95% degeneration), the end of the degeneration phase could be established with considerable precision in six (Table 3.8). In five, degeneration was complete by the 11th day at the latest, and in one patient by the 13th day at the latest. An intervening late phase involving an amplitude reduction of a few percent can be attributed, as has been discussed in some detail in Section 3.4.2, to the increasing desynchronization of compound action potential caused by progressive deceleration of speed of conduction.

Table 3.8. Zoster oticus (Groups 1 and 2)

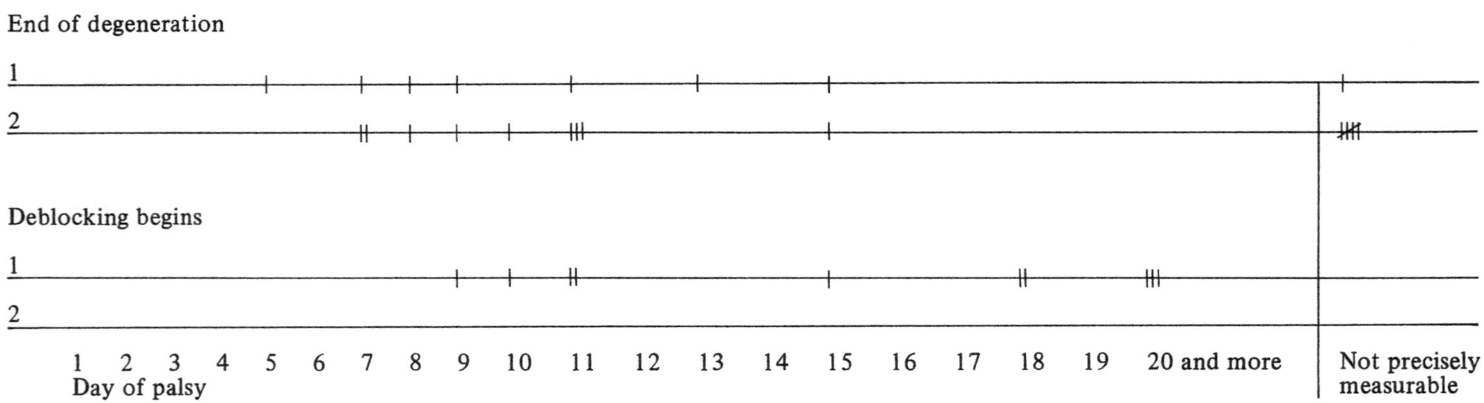

Of the nine cases in group Z2 that could provide data on this point, degeneration was complete in eight by the 11th day at the latest, by the 15th day at the latest in one other. In any case the increase in degeneration from the 11th to the 15th day was only 3%, so that even this case (Z13) does not occupy a special position.

We can therefore conclude that in the 16 measurable herpes cases the degeneration phase, on a parallel with idiopathic facial palsy, had been completed by up to the 11th day of palsy, i.e., in the light of the explanations given in Section 3.4.2 that the degenerative process at the site of the nerve lesion has come to a standstill at the 10th day of palsy.

2. Beginning of recovery from block. Group Z1 (50–95% degeneration) includes all the degrees of degeneration of groups 3 to 6 in idiopathic facial palsy. The spectrum of time values shown in Table 3.8 corresponds very well to those of groups 3 to 6.

Group Z2 includes all degrees of degeneration of groups 7 to 8 with idiopathic facial palsy. Only 3 of the total of 14 cases registered incomplete degeneration. In these 3 the beginning of recovery from block occurred at the 20th day or later—again showing complete agreement with groups 7 and 8 in idiopathic facial palsy.

This concordance is most remarkable, and leads one to suspect that in both diseases the evolution is according to principles that are essentially similar.

3. Latency. In respect to this parameter also there appears to be no essential difference from idiopathic facial palsy, so that the corresponding section on facial palsy can be referred to in the discussion.

4. End of recovery from block. Group Z1 (50–95% degeneration) shows the same spread of values (see Table 3.9) as the corresponding groups 4 to 6 in idiopathic facial palsy, i.e., axon block had completely receded between the 30th and 80th days. Any amilioration after the 80th day has to be attributed, therefore, to regeneration or reinnervation.

Table 3.9. End of deblocking

Day of palsy		20	30	40	50	60	70	80	not measurable
Case No.	Z1					x			
	Z2								x
	Z3		x						
1	Z4			x					
	Z5			x					
	Z6								x
	Z7				x				
	Z8			x					
	Z9								x
2	Z10							x	
	Z11								x

In group Z2 (95–100% degeneration) there were only three cases in which the nerve fibers did not completely degenerate. It is therefore not taken into consideration.

5. Degree of recovery of function. If we compare Table 3.10 with Table 3.4, it is clear that group Z1 (50–90% degeneration) corresponds, in regard to degree of degeneration, most closely to group 5 in idiopathic facial palsy. Since group Z1 includes the

degrees of degeneration of groups 4 to 6 in idiopathic facial palsy, the group Z1 values correspond quite closely to the middle point of these groups.

Table 3.10. Degree of regeneration in Zoster oticus

Day of palsy	60–80	90–120	180–220	300	400	500
Group: 1	13%	32%	47%			
2		2.5%	7.8%	27%	49%	

Indeed, group Z2 (95–100% degeneration), which corresponds to groups 8 and 9 in idiopathic facial palsy, also shows a surprisingly close correspondence in terms of these values with this group. *Therefore no systematic distinction can be made in the evolution of regeneration between idiopathic facial palsy and herpes oticus.*

6. Degree of functional recovery. It was possible to keep the seven cases in group Z1 under observation for long enough (until after the 200th day) to form a valid opinion of the degree of functional recovery. If the degree of degeneration in these seven cases is taken as a basis (1 x 50%, 1 x 60%, 2 x 85%, 2 x 90%, 1 x 95%), they must for purposes of comparison be ranked between groups 5 and 6 in idiopathic facial palsy. In group 5 (70–90% restitution) 23 of the 32 patients achieved full functional recovery, but in group 6 only 5 of 11. In group Z1 it was 4 out of 7. It is very likely that a longer period of examination would have brought the results much closer to those of group 5.

In 8 of the total 13 patients in group Z2 it was possible to maintain observation for quite a long period (up to 500 days). Only 2 achieved a recovery of function that could be called either good or satisfactory (Z9, Z19). In the others it ranged from unsatisfactory to poor or very poor. All those with poor or very poor functional recovery showed noticeable, and often marked, associated movement as well as facial contracture on occasion.

7. Correlation of age and degree of denervation/degree of functional recovery. The average age of all 21 herpes cases was 44.4 years. In group Z1 it was 40.7 years, and in Z2 49.9 years.

Table 3.12 sets out the average degree of degeneration of the eight youngest and eight eldest herpes cases on the 20th, 70th, and 100th days of palsy. The average age in Z1 was 31.5 years, and in Z2 58.2 years. The difference is equally as clear as in Table 3.7 for idiopathic facial palsy.

On the other hand, the difference in average age is not so marked as in idiopathic faci palsy when a comparison is made between the seven cases with best functional recovery and the seven with the worst, as is shown in Table 3.13.

Case Z14, aged 21, falls in the second column of this table. The patient, a female, admittedly showed an amplitude increase from 0% to 60% of the initial value, which corresponds to a degeneration of 40%. The clinical result did not correspond in any way, however, with this good degree of regeneration, because the patient showed particularly marked associated movement. The synkinesis was so strong that the perioral muscles were strongly innervated when she closed her eyelids, but not by the normal voluntary movements. There was similar difficulty in innervating the other facial muscles normally, so that the degree of functional recovery even at the 500th day was only 20%. It is thus evident that even in young patients misdirection by the regenerating axons can nullify the quantitatively good regeneration of nerve fibers.

Table 3.11. Degree of restitution in facial palsy

Day of palsy		30	40	50	60	70	80	90	100	120	140	160	180	200	300	400	500	600
Case No.	Z1								50					70				
	Z2										100							
	Z3										100							
1	Z4										70			80				
	Z5					100												
	Z6								60		90							
	Z8									40				40				
	Z9													70	80		95	
	Z10									20				40			65	
2	Z13													10	15			
	Z14													20		20	20	
	Z15													15	20	30		
	Z19																80	
	Z21												10			30		

Table 3.12. Average degree of degeneration of the eight youngest and eight eldest herpes oticus patients

Day of palsy	20		70		100	
Age group	1	2	1	2	1	2
	50	85	50	56	50	43
	57	88	15	92	0	92
	80	92	69	84	60	77
	90	93	58	97	50	97
	96	98	96	98	95	95
	100	100	99	100	98	100
	100	100	99	100	98	100
	100	100	100	100	99	100
	673	756	586	727	550	702
Average degree of degeneration (%)	84.1	94.5	73.2	90.8	68.7	87.7
Average age (years)	31.5	58.2				
Percent in favor of age group 1	11.1		19.4		21.3	

Table 3.13

No.	Age of patient with best functional recovery	Age of patients with worst functional recovery
1	22	21
2	29	31
3	29	47
4	42	55
5	51	65
6	53	65
7	55	76
	280	350
Average age (years)	40.0	50.0

3.4.5. Bilateral Facial Palsies: Case Reports

Case Bl: J. J., male 21 years. Beginning May 1973 severe headaches, particularly affecting temporoparietal, right. Strong lacrimation, slight burning of both eyes. Depressed, tired. On 5/8/73 an exacerbation of the headaches, facial palsy right. From 5/10/73 an improvement of the headaches. On 5/15/73 retroauricular pains, left side. Facial palsy right clearly receding. 5/16/73 facial palsy on left. From 5/23/74 facial palsy on left also receding. From 5/25/73 renewed severe headaches, most severe over the mastoid bilaterally, tinnitus, loss of hearing, more marked on right than on left. X-ray on 5/29/73. CSF 5/29/73: clear, colorless, total proteins 39 mg%, 104/3 cell count (76% lymphocytes, 24% reticulum cells). CFS check on 6/8/73: Protein 46 mg%, 346/3 cells (93% lymphocytes, 7% reticulum cells). SR 8 mm, leucocytes 9200, white cell picture unremarkable, virus serology negative. Later history: Headaches continuing until autumn 1973. Clinically complete recovery from facial palsy and hearing disturbance by end August 1973.
Diagnosis: Bilateral facial palsy and cochlearis involvement, with lymphocytic meningitis, probably of viral etiology.

Case B2: N. S., male 13 years. Beginning April 1972 swelling over left mastoid apparently after insect bite. On 4/12/72 facial palsy on left. 4/14/72 otological examination unremarkable. Leucocytes 4050. Smear unremarkable. 4/19/72 multiple cervical lymph gland swellings, with isolated swellings nuchal and axillary, left. Because of general worsening of condition hospitalization from 4/26/72 to 5/5/72. Status 4/26/72: Generally below par, neck stiffness, throbbing left side of head, Lasègue positive at 70 °. Submandibular and nuchal painfulness bilaterally, lymphatic nodosities size of hazel-nut. CSF: protein 127 mg %, cell count: 230 mononuclear, 24 polynuclear, and 37 macrophage. Further evolution: As facial palsy began to recede on left, facial palsy began on right on 4/28/72. CSF on 4/20/72: obvious change for the better: protein 100 mg %, 5 mononuclear. Clinically complete recovery from palsy by November 1973.
Diagnosis: Bilateral facial palsy with lymphocytic meningitis, apparently of viral origin.

Case B3: G. A., male, 68 years. Arthritic episodes in knee and hip joint, left, with recurrence over period of 30 years. May 1973 a renewed attack. Beginning of June headaches lasting several days, slight meningism, accompanied by taste disturbance, particularly on left half of tongue. Chewing weakness. Wife noticed a decline in alertness. Gradual improvement until mid-July. On 7/14/73 facial palsy began right, and on 7/21/73 also on left. Hospitalization from 7/31/73 to 8/8/73. Condition on 7/30/73: Bilateral facial palsy, but not total, right somewhat more severe than left. Hypogeusia of right half of tongue. General mental decline. Disturbance of memory. EMG: no denervation potentials: Fairly numerous active motor units. Degree of degeneration right 55%, left 50%. Serum (3.8): Protein 35 mg %, Cell count 104/3 (93% lymphocytes, 7% reticulum cells). Serum check on 10.8: protein 32 mg %, cell count 88/3 (91% lymphocytes, 8% reticulum cells, 1% plasma cells). Leuco 12 800, distribution unremarkable. For evolution see graph.
Diagnosis: Bilateral facial palsy with lymphocytic meningitis, probably of viral etiology.

Case B4: E. S., male, 46 years. From beginning of August 1974 pains in left thorax and arm. On 8/25/74 on wakening found bilateral facial palsy. Position on 8/26/74: complete palsy bilaterally. Sense of taste affected. Some active motor units shown by EMG. Compound action potential right 3200 μV left 2200 μV. As initial value is not known, an average of 5500 μV is taken as a basis. End of degeneration at about 65% bilaterally on 9th day of palsy (see graph). Rapid disappearance of chest pain. A proposed hospitalization and CSF check could not be carried out for external reasons.
Diagnosis: Bilateral facial palsy with polyradiculitis was assumed, in connection with preceding pain in thorax and arm lasting about a week (see case B6).

Case B5: P. B., male, 43 years. Since 1967 a history of episodes, lasting from a week to a month, of heat and formication paresthesia in both hands and on right side of face. Serum test 1968 without anything remarkable. Diagnosis of suspected multiple sclerosis. Since 11/26/72 headaches, dysesthesia and paresthesia in hands and feet. On 12/2/62 facial palsy bilaterally, and numbness on right cheek. Hospitalization from 12/5/72 to 12/15/72. Findings: Total facial palsy bilaterally. Sense of taste greatly reduced. Glove and sock-type hypoesthesia of hands and feet. CSF: protein 94 mg %, cell count 4/3 (lymphocytes 73%, monocytes 21%, neutrophils 1%, reticulum cells 5%). EMG on 12/7/72: Complete bilateral loss of innervation of facial muscles. Degeneration degree right 60%, left 80% (see diagram). Slight reduction of impulse conduction speed in ulnar nerve (45 m/s). Leucoc. 8900, normal distribution. EMG (12/11/72). Nothing notable. Further evolution: Headaches and dysesthesia receded in course of 2 months. Beginning of recovery from facial palsy could be recognized from 1/10/73. Up to October 1973 retreat of palsy to 50%, no facial asymmetry. Synkinesis.
Diagnosis: Bilateral facial palsy with polyradiculitis.

Case B6: A. S., male, 52 years. From end 1973 chest pains in form of bands, particularly on left side, dysesthesia of left half of thorax. On 2/23/74 facial palsy right. Hospitalization from 2/25/74 to 4/4/74. Dysesthesia and hypoesthesia of hands and feet. From 2/25/74 prednisolone therapy, 60 mg/d. On 2/28/74 facial palsy left. CSF: protein 43 mg%, 18/3 cells (mononuclear). CSF check on 3/18/74: protein 52 mg%, 33/3 cells, of which 18/3 mononuclear. EMG: Intercostal muscles, right; considerable denervation. Oblique muscle of abdomen, right: Denervation potentials. Trunc. erector, both sides: Denervation potentials. Speed of conduction tibial nerve: 36m/s. Loss of vital capacity up to 1.5 l. Degeneration of the facial nerve of up to over 99% (see graph). After a transitory improvement of the general condition, a further relapse in May.

Increased pain and disturbance of sensation in arms and legs, increased unsteadiness of gait, reduced sensitivity to vibration. EMG of 6/5/74: Short flexor muscle of great toe: Plentiful denervation potentials, marked deficit in activity of motor units. Marked dispersion of compound action potential on stimulation of tibial nerve. Conduction velocity 34 m/s. In July and August a gradual general improvement. On 2/3/74 a slight mimetic innervation detectable bilaterally. Development of bilateral facial contracture, so that the patient can no longer close lips. Slight unsteadiness of gait continues. Position sense and vibration sense improved. EMG shows no new denervation. Speed of conduction, tibial nerve still 34 m/s.
Diagnosis: Bilateral facial palsy with recurring polyradiculitis.

Case B7: E. S., female, 50 years. On 5/30/72 appearance of facial palsy on right without preliminary symptoms. First examination on third day of palsy. Findings: Subtotal facial palsy right, infra-auricular neuralgia right, no disturbance of taste. EMG: a number of active motor units. 50% degree of degeneration of facial nerve. Evolution: degeneration ends on 6/7/72, beginning of block recovery from 6/15/72. Good progress until 8/24/72 (see graph). On 8/25/72 on rising patient notices facial palsy on left. No preliminary symptoms. On the same day burning in left eye, feeling of numbness on left side of face. Findings on 8/28/72: total palsy on left side of face, ageusia. EMG: no active motor units. Compound action potential loss of 44% of original value. Evolution (see graph): Degeneration up to 90%. End of degeneration on 8th day of palsy. Beginning of recovery from block about the 20th day.
Diagnosis: Idiopathic facial palsy first on the right, then on the left.

Case B8: N. H., female, 53 years. During the night of 6/24/72 headache left side. On 9/24/72 no taste on left half of tongue. In the evening feeling of tightness in left cheek, lacrimation of left eye, facial weakness on that side. 9/26/72: Complete loss of innervation of facial muscles, left side, ageusia left half of tongue. In the days following infra-auricular neuralgia on left gradually receding. Facial palsy receding from 10/20/72. On 10/19/72 headache, infra-auricular neuralgia right. On 10/20/72 dysesthesia on right half of face, onset of facial palsy. No taste on right half of tongue. Facial palsy of right side receding from 10/21/72.
Diagnosis: Bilateral facial palsy of unexplained etiology, possibly idiopathic facial palsy.

3.4.6. Bilateral Facial Palsies: Principles of Evolution

This group includes facial palsies of different etiologies (cf., section 1.2.3): three cases of lymphocytic meningitis (B1–3), three cases of polyradiculitis (B4–6), and two cases where the etiology was not established (B7–8).

The eight cases dealt with do not show any notable divergence from the seven parameters within which we have already discussed the evolution of both idiopathic facial palsy and herpes oticus. Degeneration was complete within the first 10–11 days, and where that did not appear to be the case (B2 and B6), it must be emphasized that there were not enough points of measurement to present an accurate picture. As before, the beginning of recovery from block was related to the severity of degeneration, and regeneration and recovery of function followed the lines already indicated.

There is good reason, however, to give this group a special section, because of the possibility that arose here to make use of the methodology as described to make an exact comparison of the evolution of the disease on both sides. This has never been done before.

1. Bilateral Facial Palsy in Lymphocytic Meningitis

Information is scanty about the pathogenesis of facial palsy in association with a lymphocytic meningitis. Among the few things we know is that there is inflammation of the meninges, particularly the arachnoidea, with a rise in the pressure of the cerebrospinal fluid and increased cell count (lymphocytes, plasma cells). The process can extend through the vessels until it reaches the cerebral parenchyma (meningoencephalitis). As was explained in section 1.1.1, the cerebrospinal fluid cavity branches off to accompany the facial nerve into the internal auditory meatus, and in some patients continues for a few millimeters into the facial canal. It can be assumed that the facial nerve is affected at the point of the cerebrospinal fluid cavity where there is usually a narrow section, i.e., at the entrance to the fallopian canal. Moreover, it is clearly not affected simply by the rise in CSF pressure, otherwise we would encounter facial palsies much more frequently in all cases of increase of intracranial pressure. But it is possible that the rise in pressure and congestion at the entrance to the facial canal assists the pathogenic agent (probably viral) to pass from the fluid to the nerve sheath. This could trigger pathogenetic processes of the type that can be observed in both idiopathic facial palsy and herpes oticus. The fact that the degeneration and regeneration phases evolve over similar time periods would strongly support such an assumption.

A study of the case profiles of B1, B2, and B3 brings out at once the remarkable similarity between the amplitude, latency, and palsy (or recovery) curves. In order to show that maximal degeneration and palsy is reached in each patient completely bilaterally, it is simply a matter of adding a few days to the time periods for degeneration, recovery from block, and regeneration. It is instructive to make a closer analysis of the curves of the individual cases:

B1: The palsy began suddenly on the right side after a preliminary period of at least a week of feeling ill with headache on the right side. The first evaluation was carried out on the 2nd day of palsy. On that day it was still not possible to detect any difference in amplitude between the two sides of the face. A degree of degeneration of 24% was reached on the 7th day of palsy, and at the same time the palsy (the axon block) clearly began to recede. On the 9th day of palsy paralysis set in suddenly on the left side, even though the patient had been having prednisolone therapy (30 mg daily) since the day of palsy onset. The palsy on the left side was evaluated from its day of onset, when it already showed a degree of degeneration of 14%. Within the next 2 days it fell to 36%, and then stabilized. At the same time there was a further slight fall in amplitude on the right side, i.e., between the 9th and 11th days of palsy, after the compound action potential had shown a degree of degeneration of 24% for a full day. There was a further degeneration of 12% between the 9th and 11th days, so that by the 11th day on the right, and the 3rd day on the left, the facial nerve showed equal degeneration bilaterally. Axon block disappeared quite rapidly on both sides, although it lagged for a few days on the left.

Two main inferences can be drawn from this history: (1) the fact that the compound action potential on the left side of the face indicated degeneration of a part of the nerve fibers on the day of palsy onset is evidence that for some time previously the disease was already present. However, it was slower to become manifest than the palsy affecting the right side. We can conclude that what might be termed the "date of illness" of both nerves was much closer than "date of appearance". Furthermore, the disease process followed a less acute course on the left than on the right. (2) Even though the "time constant" for the disease process was somewhat different between the sides, there was no difference in the severity of the affection as such. The overall impression is that this parameter of severity, i.e., the definitive extent of nerve fiber degeneration, has already been established even before the palsy makes itself manifest. This view is strengthened by the evident ineffectiveness of the drug prednisolone, which had been prescribed from the 2nd day of palsy on the right side. It could be speculated that although the drug delayed the outbreak of palsy on the left side, it could not materially affect the process of damage to the nerve. Against this, however, it should be mentioned that at the very point when the degeneration phase was reaching completion on the left side, a second mild wave of degeneration was observable on the right. This could be a hint that some days previously there had been an exacerbation of the illness. Since recovery from block was detectable on the right side as early as the 7th day of palsy, it must be assumed that this sudden exacerbation had come to an end at least one to two days before.

B2: In this case the time interval between the appearance of palsy on the left side, first of all, and then on the right, was 18 days, longer than in B1. Nevertheless, the degeneration and regeneration curves bilaterally were very similar. It is probable that the resemblance would have been even closer if more values had been entered during the period between the 10th and 20th days of palsy. This was for external reasons simply not possible, and since the records with the details of the degree of palsy during the first 20 days were also mislaid, the palsy and recovery graphs could not be drawn.

B3: The paresis began first on the right, and 7 days later appeared on the left side. The patient presented relatively late for the first examination, i.e., on the 17th day of palsy on the right, and on the 10th day of palsy on the left. For this reason it was not possible to measure the amplitude at outset. A value of 6000 μV was set arbitrarily. This is an admissible procedure for the purpose of making comparisons of the two sides, and evaluating the course of the disease. Naturally there is no way of saying in such circumstances whether maximal degeneration reached a point 10% higher or lower than appears on the chart, but since this drawback applies bilaterally, their relative difference is not misrepresented. Since the divergence or convergence of the chart curves is the main point in this discussion of the bilateral palsy group, case B3 can certainly be included.

2. Bilateral Facial Palsy with Polyradiculitis

In both B4 and B5 facial palsy began bilaterally on the same day. In these two cases it was also not possible to establish the normal value for the amplitude of the compound action potential. An arbitrary value at outset of 5500 μV was taken as a basis—corresponding to the average value (see 3.1.0: Compound action potential). If the actual value had been higher or lower, the only consequence would have been a corresponding shift of the amplitude curve either upwards or downwards, which would be the same for both sides. This would not affect the comparison between the curves, however.

B4: Degeneration had been completed bilaterally on the 9th day. At this point the amplitude curves were only showing a variance of about 6%. This divergence did not affect the clinically observable degree of palsy. Much more important during the whole period was the complete symmetry of facial innervation, i.e., from the 2nd to the 4th day of palsy complete loss of function of the facial muscles, and from the 6th day on an equally rapid recovery from axon block.

B5: Here too the paresis set in bilaterally on the same day. On the 10th day of palsy there was about 90% degeneration on both sides, and the amplitude curves were only showing about 4% divergence. A further slight loss of amplitude could be observed between the 10th and 20th days of palsy, which could be attributed for the most part to increasing desynchronization of compound action potential. The role of desynchronization is strongly attested by the sharp increase of latency (i.e., slowing of conduction velocity) up to the 20th day of palsy. At this time the amplitude curves were diverging by only about 2%. The regeneration and recovery curves continued to evolve more or less in unison. On the 300th day of palsy both nerves had the same degree of regeneration, and both sides of the face the same degree of recovery of function. The clinical end result was materially affected, however, by associated movement, recognizable from the narrow separation between the regeneration and recovery curves (cf. 3.4.2.6).

B6: Palsy appeared on the left side 5 days after it had appeared on the right, and in this case the value of compound action potential amplitude could be established at onset. The left facial nerve showed a degree of degeneration on the 2nd day of palsy of 18%. The 1st day of palsy on the left corresponded to the 6th day of palsy on the right. It is noteworthy that at the point in time when the palsy on the left appeared, there was a sharp fall in amplitude of about 69% on the right between the 5th and 7th days of palsy. As already seen in B1 (and B2) the amplitude curve of the nerve first affected by paresis falls more steeply than the one where palsy came later, even though the definitive extent of degeneration is in both cases identical. It is also noteworthy that the fall in amplitude in B1 and B6 corresponds to the appearance of paralysis on the opposing side–an indication that the relevant pathogenetic events were exacerbated in the 2 preceding days.

A final point to bear in mind with regard to B6 is the sharp increase of latency between the 6th and 20th days of palsy, which resembles the pattern seen in B4. Very possibly a marked prolongation of latency frequently occurs in facial palsy associated with polyradiculitis.

B7: In this 50-year-old patient there was a 3-month interval between the appearance of palsy first on the right side and then on the left. There were no additional symptoms that might have indicated a lymphocytic meningitis or a polyradiculitis. Yet it seems hardly likely that the palsies on both sides can be attributed to the same event. The curves for both sides also show a much greater divergence than was seen in cases B1–B6.

The fact that the etiology remained so unclear strengthens the hypothesis that this was a truly idiopathic facial palsy, with onset first on the right, and then on the left, during a period of heightened susceptibility.

B8: In this case the palsy on the right side appeared 26 days after onset on the left. At this point in time recovery from block on the left side was already in full swing, so no further increase in degeneration could be observed. For that reason also it is questionable whether this bilateral facial palsy represents a single disease event of the type seen in cases B1–B6. In any case, there was closer congruence between the curves than in case B7, even if it was still less than in cases B1–B6.

To sum up, we can make the following generalizations from this review of the bilateral facial palsies (cf. Tables 3.14, 3.15):

Table 3.14. End of deblocking

Day of palsy		20	30	40	50	60	70	80	Not measurable
Case									
B1	R	x							
	L	x							
B3	R		x						
	L		x						
B4	R		x						
	L		x						
B5	R			x					
	L			x					
B7	R		x						
	L			x					
B8	R		x						
	L		x						

Table 3.15. Degree of regeneration in bilateral facial palsy

Day of palsy	60–80		90–120		180–220		300		400		500	
Case	R	L	R	L	R	L	R	L	R	L	R	L
B1	7	15	36	36								
B2	34	32			72	72						
B3			37	40								
B4	12	10										
B5			5	5	26	20	44	50				
B6					0	6						
B7			24	34					64	52		
B8	8	16			14	31						

1. When bilateral facial palsy occurs in conjunction with an underlying illness (lymphocytic meningitis, polyradiculitis), the history on both sides from the end point of degeneration is remarkably similar. However, the amplitude curve shows a steeper fall on that side where the palsy first occurs (and degeneration tends to be more acute).

2. Prolongation of the latency is much more marked in polyradiculitis than in lymphocytic meningitis. This would point to a much more severe axonal lesion in polyradiculitis (cf. 3.4.2.3).

3. The time periods for degeneration and regeneration, for the beginning and end of recovery from block and also for recovery of function, correspond to the basic principles already formulated for idiopathic facial palsy.

3.4.7. Acute Facial Palsies of Different Etiologies

In this group we bring together the histories and brief clinical data of eight cases of unilateral facial paresis with known, but differing etiology (that is, where there was a different, but identifiable underlying illness). This group was included in the study in order to extend the possibilities of comparison with the other groups.

The following were the individual diagnoses:

V1: Facial palsy associated with lymphocytic meningitis
V2: Facial palsy with polyradiculitis
V3: Facial palsy in Melkersson-Rosenthal syndrome
V4: Facial palsy following surgical intervention (heat lesion of nerve during cauterization)
V5: Facial palsy in otitis media
V6: Facial palsy associated with a translabyrinthine operation on an acoustic nerve neurinome
V7: Facial palsy in hypoliquorrhea syndrome
V8: Chronic progressive facial palsy in association with epithelial carcinoma of the parotid gland

Apart from V8, this was a series of "acute" facial palsies. It seemed useful, however, if only for contrast, to include at least one case of chronic progressive palsy, since in these, too, there are important advantages in electroneurography. Such palsies progress so slowly that it is often quite difficult to make a judgement solely on the basis of clinical observation. Furthermore, a clinical estimation of the full extent of nerve fiber degeneration is not infrequently erroneous. In some of these chronic cases the part played by axon block in the paresis can be quite limited, and a much greater role is assumed by nerve fiber degeneration. As was pointed out already in Section 3.4.2.4, there has to be a deficiency of 50% or more of facial motor fibers before palsy becomes clinically observable.

Thus even a palsy that looks only moderate can quite often–to the physician's surprise–have already reached a degree of degeneration of 80–90%. But when electroneurographic techniques are used, the degree of degeneration can be measured from the 1st day of examination onward, and further checks clearly show any increasing degeneration.

Cases V1 and V2 correspond to cases B1–3, and B4–6 respectively, and offer nothing essentially different. They have been included here because they offer models for unilateral facial palsy with lymphatic meningitis or with polyradiculitis. In both cases the evolution was quite benign, with nothing distinguishable from the histories of idiopathic facial palsy in groups 2 and 3.

Of this group, V3 is an example of a Melkersson-Rosenthal syndrome. As indicated already in Section 2.1.2, transtemporal decompression was carried out in two patients with this syndrome (cf. also Table 2.3). In both cases the operation microscope showed findings similar to an idiopathic facial palsy, i.e., swelling and hemorrhagia of the nerve in the fundus of the acoustic meatus and strangulation at the entry to the facial canal. Only in this case was it possible to make some attempt at making a graph of evolution, and even then it was very fragmentary, with a great deal missing at the beginning and end.

Case V4 was an iatrogenic facial palsy associated with a radical operation. The facial palsy was recognizable immediately after the operation and was attributed to the effect of heat from cauterization in a site near the nerve. Thus quite involuntarily a situation developed which corresponded to the animal experiment by Boyle (1967). (Compare Section 1.2.1.)

The patient, a female, came for the first examination on the 5th day of palsy. Degeneration was calculated at 74%. It was also evident that by far the greater part of the fibers damaged irreversibly by heat had already degenerated. A secondary edema, corresponding to a secondary ischemia, had ensued, but did not seem to have played a significant part with regard to the degree of nerve damage. The following reasons can be advanced for this opinion: (1) the facial palsy on the 5th day of palsy was not total (and in the opinion of the operator had not been total before). An edema which had caused degeneration of three-quarters of the motor fibers would in any case have blocked the rest, including those that had not degenerated. And since the palsy was not complete, not all the fibers had been blocked. On the basis of the experience gained in analyzing many graphs of idiopathic facial palsy and herpes oticus it seems more probable to calculate that of the 25% of fibers remaining that had not degenerated by the 5th day after palsy onset only about half were blocked. (2) Even in severe cases, including considerable edema and corresponding strangulation, degeneration is scarcely complete on the 5th day of palsy. In the present case only a bare 12% further decline in amplitude of the compound action potential was recorded between the 5th and 12th days of palsy, and the marked prolongation of latency indicates a growing deceleration of the impulse conduction, i.e., a desynchronization of the compound action potential. This goes a long way to explain the slowness of the phase of amplitude reduction. (3) It is also unusual that the palsy should not be total, in spite of the marked prolongation of latency to almost double the value at outset. No analogy exists for this in idiopathic facial palsy or in the herpes cases. It must be concluded that the axonal lesion that causes the slowing of impulse conduction should be attributed to a large extent to the heat damage rather than to the edema and consequent ischemia.

The later evolution was marked by rapid regeneration and recovery of function, which in fact also corresponds with the findings in Boyle's animal experiments. The connective tissue of the nerve, and the endoneurium in particular, seems to have been less affected by the heat than the more sensitive axons.

V5 is representative of the evolution of a facial palsy associated with otitis media. Four days before the appearance of palsy there was acute onset of otitis media. At the first examination on the 4th day of palsy (9th day of otitis), the degeneration phase which had reached 56% was already completed, as the later evolution showed. The lesion had doubtless already been operative in the nerve for several days before the palsy actually appeared, but the degenerative process was quickly halted by the paracentesis, which rapidly afforded relief, and the beginning of antibiotic therapy. The later history indicated a very rapid and very satisfactory regeneration and functional recovery. The fact that the latency remained constant points to an absence of "axonal disease".

Case V6 can be regarded as an iatrogenic facial palsy which was in a way unavoidable. Paralysis of the nerve set in immediately after a very carefully executed translabyrinthine detachment of the facial nerve from an acoustic nerve neurinome, carried out under the microscope. By the 8th day of palsy degeneration of 98% of all fibers had already been completed. In spite of fairly good regeneration, the functional result at the 450th day remained poor–and definitively so–as a result of severe associated movement and facial contracture.

It would have been of great interest to have been able to follow the evolution of a greater number of cases of acoustic nerve neurinome, since here both the time point and the point of lesion are known with precision. Unfortunately, this was not possible.

In case V7 there was onset of facial palsy 14 days after replacement of the bone plate following a craniotomy for oligodendroglioma. The most marked clinical symptom after the operation was severe hypoliquorrhea syndrome. Whether this had any part in the etiology remains an open question. In any case the history diverged from the general trends seen in idiopathic facial palsy and herpes oticus in that recovery from block began between the 4th and 9th days of palsy, even though the process of degeneration was doubtless still continuing. It is difficult to say whether any hard and fast conclusions can be drawn about the relevant pathogenetic events in this case. However, it would not seem very likely, judging from the graph, that there was edema and strangulation of the nerve at the entry to the facial canal.

V8 presents the profile one would expect from a chronic, progressive facial palsy. The patient, a female, presented for the first examination 16 days after experiencing facial weakness. It seems very probable that the palsy, which increased gradually in the days following, had already set in some considerable time beforehand. The first review on the 22nd day of palsy indicated no change. On the 28th day a further increase in degeneration as well as of the degree of palsy, could be observed, and both continued to increase until the 33rd day. In view of the unusual evolution, the patient was subjected to a detailed otologic examination, which led to the discovery of an epithelial carcinoma of the parotid gland.

To summarize, we can conclude that, in regard to the evolution of the degeneration and paresis curves, cases V1, V2 and probably also V3, present nothing unusual as compared to the curves seen in idiopathic facial palsy. On the other hand, some divergences can be seen in cases V4, V5, and V7. In all likelihood this would also have applied to case V6, if the first examination had been carried out soon enough. Nevertheless, it can be assumed that in this case degeneration was already completed by the 2nd or 3rd day of palsy. Case V8 falls completely outside the rest of the series of profiles presented here.

3.4.8. Facial Palsies in Petrosal Bone Fractures

Where facial palsy is due to trauma it is difficult as a rule to begin recording the natural history profile with any exactitude within the first 10 days. This is because petrosal bone fractures are frequently accompanied by loss of consciousness, and during the early days the patient is usually lying in an apathetic condition in the emergency ward. At that stage observation is not directed to the facial palsy. As a consequence it is often impossible to obtain reliable data concerning the point in time when the palsy first shows itself. This lack of precision applies in particular to the so-called late phase, which supervenes from a few days to two weeks after the accident, and during which the palsy becomes visible.

It is well known that transverse fractures of the pyramid lead more frequently to facial palsy and cause greater damage to the facial nerve in consequence than do longitudinal fractures. In the latter, the palsy is caused not so much by direct trauma to the nerve, as by the fact that edema and blood seepage in the region of the canal and the nerve sheath lead in the course of a few days to axon block and degeneration. This can involve a considerable portion of the nerve fibers.

The case profiles of six late palsies of this type, associated with radiologically demonstrated longitudinal pyramidal fractures, are, briefly, as follows:

In case T1 the degeneration was already receding on the 4th day of palsy (1st day of examination), in case T2 on the 6th day of palsy. Degeneration was completed at the latest by the 12th day of palsy in T3. However, values are missing between the 7th and 12th day of palsy, so it is conceivable that degeneration had already ended at an earlier point in time. In cases T4–6 the patients presented so late for examination that it was not possible to measure the course of degeneration with any accuracy.

On the other hand, there were sufficient data in all cases from which to make judgements concerning nerve fiber regeneration and recovery of function. As in all other facial palsy groups, these parameters are clearly linked with the degree of severity of degeneration. Thus, in cases T2 and T6, in which all motor fibers degenerated, functional recovery was either poor or very poor. The T2 profile shows that the amplitude and recovery curves intersect on the 260th day of palsy, which, as seen earlier, is a certain sign of misdirection and corresponding associated movement. This is to be blamed for the poor result. In the other cases recovery of function ranged from good to very good, even in case T5 with degeneration of 91%. We can conclude from this, even though the group was relatively small, that in all likelihood the processes of regeneration and functional recovery in traumatic facial palsy obey principles similar to those that apply in the idiopathic and other groups.

3.5. Prognosis of Acute Facial Palsies

There is little difficulty in establishing the main principles for prognosis in the facial palsy groups dealt with here, if we take as a basis the evidence assembled in Sections 3.4.2 to 3.4.8 combined with systematic comparison of the natural history profile. These principles can be set out in tabular form. Apart from the insight gained from the analysis of more than 100 case profiles, the most important conclusions to emerge is that nerve fiber degeneration as measured by electroneurography is completed at the latest by the 10th to the 12th day of palsy.

1. The prognosis is invariably good if degeneration of the facial nerve fibers has not exceeded 90%.

2. The prognosis is good in the greater majority of cases if degeneration of the facial nerve fibers does not exceed 95%.

3. Where the degree of degeneration is from 95–98%, functional recovery ranging from satisfactory to very good can be expected in one case in two, although the recovery phase can extend to more than 300 days.

4. If the degree of degeneration exceeds 98%, the prognosis is uncertain. However, good recovery of function is possible in individual cases even where degeneration has been 100%.

Rules 1–4 constitute a basis for prognosis of facial palsy without taking the time factor into consideration. If it is necessary to express an opinion concerning the amount of time likely to elapse between the 1st day of palsy and good recovery of function, the following rules can be established:

5. There will be good functional recovery of the facial muscles within 4 weeks if the degree of degeneration is below 10% by the 10th day of palsy.

6. There will be good or very good recovery of function by the paralysed face muscles in 4–6 weeks if the degree of degeneration is under 50% on the 10th day of palsy.

7. The recovery of function will be good to very good in 6–10 weeks if the degree of degeneration is under 70% on the 10th day of palsy.

8. If a level of 90% degeneration had been reached on the day of palsy, good return of function will require a period of 4 months or more.

9. Where the degree of degeneration is over 95% good recovery of function will take more than 6 months–if it is achieved at all.

Rules 1 to 9 enable the physician to make a reliable prognosis in over 95% of patients by the 12th day of palsy at the latest, and often much earlier. In at least 80% of patients a reliable predication can be made concerning the degree of recovery of function even by the end of the 1st week.

10. If degeneration has not exceeded 30% by up to the 6th day of palsy, good recovery of function within 6 weeks can be predicted. The same applies if degeneration has not exceeded 40% by the 8th day.

It is not normally possible to make a reliable prognostic statement before the 4th day of palsy, unless by that time a level of degeneration of 50% has already been exceeded. In the latter circumstances, the prognosis is either poor or doubtful. On the other hand, if there has been little or no detectable degeneration by the 4th day the situation is essentially unpredictable. This is because in a large number of cases the degeneration gradient falls most steeply after the 4th day.

The most important rules for prognosis are presented in summarized form in the following table.

Table 3.16. Dependence of prognosis on degree of degeneration and day of palsy

Day of palsy	4	6	8	10	12
Degree of degeneration (%)					
< 30	+				
< 40	(+)	+			
< 50	?	(+)			
< 60		?	+		
< 70			(+)		
< 80			?	+	
< 90				(+)	+
< 95				?	(+)
> 95					?

\+ = good prognosis
(+) = probably good
? = doubtful or poor

3.6. Operation in Acute Facial Palsy: Transtemporal Decompression

Dr. U. Fisch had up to December 1974 carried out transtemporal decompression on 25 patients for idiopathic facial palsy, herpes oticus and Melkerson-Rosenthal syndrome. A profile of the case history could be established in 15 of these patients, including 11 in which it covered all phases. In the other 4 it was either in the opening, middle, or late phase. On 13 occasions the operation was carried out before the 10th day of palsy, as the following tabulation shows:

Day of palsy:	2	3	4	5	6	7	8	9	10
Cases:	1		1	1	1	2	4	3	

In one case the operation was carried out on the 28th day, and in one case on the 33rd day.

In the first part of this work all those cases were tabulated (2.1 to 2.3) in which either intratemporal stimulation was performed and/or a preoperative or postoperative case profile could be established. In the section that follows here only those cases will be evaluated in which it was possible to draw up a case profile based on electroneurographic findings.

The following cases were taken into consideration for the evaluation:

1. 5 cases of idiopathic facial palsy (80, 117, 129, 131, 140), (see Fig. 14).

2. 9 cases of herpes oticus (Z3, 4, 8, 10, 12, 14, 16, 17, 19), (see Fig. 15 for those cases in which postoperatively the degeneration phase was not complete, and Fig. 16 for those in which degeneration was either complete preoperatively or became so postoperatively)

3. 1 case of Melkersson-Rosenthal syndrome.

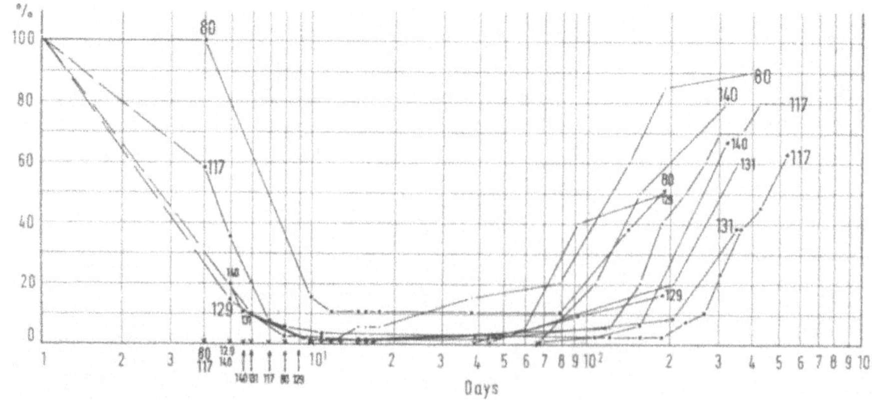

Fig. 9. Profiles of 5 cases of idiopathic facial palsy with transtemporal decompression (see text). Arrows indicate day of operation

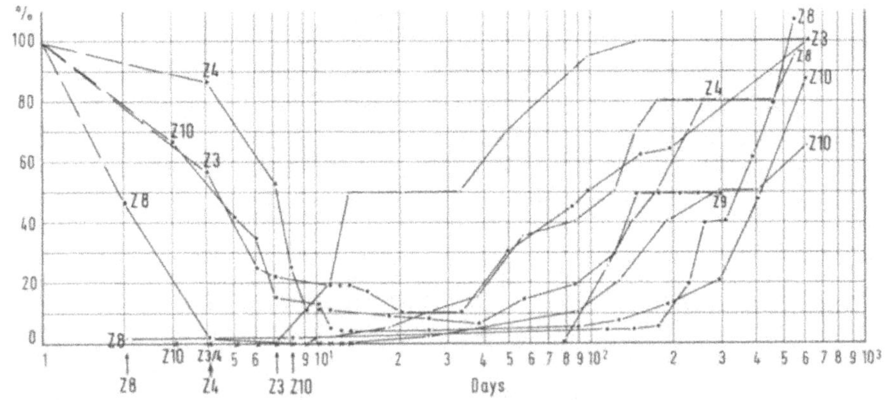

Fig. 10. Profiles of 4 cases of zoster oticus with incomplete degeneration of facial nerve at transtemporal decompression. Arrows indicate day of operation

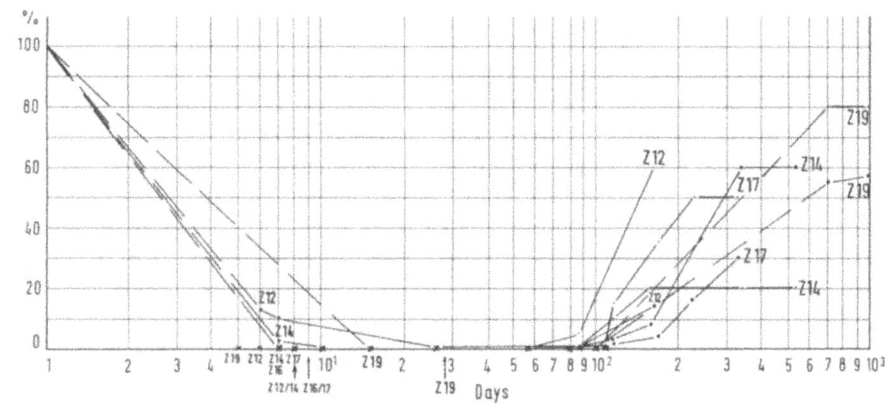

Fig. 11. Profiles of 5 cases of zoster oticus where degeneration of facial nerve was already complete at transtemporal decompression. Arrows indicate day of operation

3.6.1. Evolution of Operated Cases

A short review of the individual cases is essential for a precise analysis.

Case 80 (Table 2.1, No. 3): The transtemporal decompression was carried out on the 8th day of palsy during a phase when the degeneration gradient was very steep. Degeneration came to a halt at 90% on the 4th postoperative day, i.e., on the 12th day. It is extremely difficult to say whether this would also have been the case if the operation had not been carried out. Functional recovery was good by the 400th day.

Case 117 (Table 2.1, No. 4): The decompression was carried out on the 7th day of palsy with a degree of 93% degeneration. Thereafter only a slight decline in amplitude could be observed, which could be attributed to desynchronization of compound action potential as a result of marked slowing of conduction velocity. Satisfactory recovery of function up to the 500th day.

Case 129 (Table 2.1, No. 5): Decompression on the 9th day of palsy with 98% degeneration. The further course showed no increase in degeneration, and improvement of function and regeneration began quite early. The case is at present being surveyed up to the 200th day, but promises good recovery of function over the period 100–200th day.

Case 131 (Table 2.1, No. 6): Transtemporal decompression on the 6th day of palsy with 91% degeneration. Only slight increase of degeneration up to the 10th day. The point of "moderate" recovery of function reached by the 360th day. Further progress affected by presence of associated movement.

Case 140 (Table 2.1, No. 7): Transtemporal decompression on the evening of the 5th day of palsy with a degree of degeneration of 90%, compared with a measurement at 80% that morning. The decompression did not prevent degeneration reaching completion by up to the 10th day. Satisfactory recovery of function up to the 330th day. A favourable course when compared to the average result in group 9.

Case Z3 (Table 2.2, No. 4): Decompression on the 7th day of palsy with 78% degeneration. Amplitude stopped falling up to a late phase between the 15th and 20th days, which could be attributed to desynchronization of compound action potential following an increase of latency. Very good recovery and regeneration.

Case Z4 (Table 2.2, No. 2): Emergency decompression already on the 4th day of palsy, even though at this point degeneration could only be shown to be at 13%. The decisive factor was the involvement of vestibular and cochlear nerves as early as the 3rd day. Degeneration came to a halt at about 90% on the 9th day. The further loss of amplitude of about 5% up to the 38th day can be attributed to desynchronization of compound action potential. Satisfactory recovery of function had been achieved by the 170th day. No further improvement due to the presence of associated movement.

Case Z8 (Table 2.2, No. 3): A degree of degeneration of 53% was noted on the 1st day of examination (2nd day of palsy). An extensive herpes rash had appeared some 7 days previously on the face, neck and external ear. Since the vestibular and cochlear nerves were also involved, an emergency decompression was indicated. Degeneration rose by the 4th day to 98% and then leveled out. The patient plays the clarinet in an orchestra, and therefore practices unusually often and for long periods. At the 250th day he could again play short pieces quite well, but was not able to hold the longer notes, because his lips did not hold the mouthpiece of the instrument tightly enough to prevent air escaping. At the 400th day he could again play with the orchestra in performances. The functional end result is somewhat affected by slight associated movement and facial contracture.

Case Z10 (Table 2.2, No. 1): Transtemporal decompression on the 8th day of palsy with 85% degeneration. Involvement of vestibular and cochlear nerves. Degeneration halted on 12th day at 95%. The amplitude and palsy curves intersected on 400th day, with development of marked associated movement, clearly affecting the functional result.

Case Z12 (Table 2.2, No. 8): Transtemporal decompression on 8th day of palsy with a degeneration of over 90%. A postoperative examination on the 26th day (for external reasons earlier examination was not possible) revealed complete degeneration.

Probably all facial nerve fibers had already degenerated by the 10th to the 12th day. Beginning of regeneration and functional recovery observed at about the 90th day, and was unusually well advanced by the 165th day. However, a relatively quite marked associated movement also supervened, so it is not certain whether the end result will reach the level of "good to very good".

Case Z14 (Table 2.2, No. 6): Transtemporal decompression on 8th day of palsy with degeneration almost complete. Involvement of vestibular and cochlear nerves. Complete degeneration of all facial nerve motor fibers noted by 10th day. Quite good regeneration up to the 350th day. Functional improvement after good progress stopped completely from 160th day, because of development of extremely strong associated movement and facial contracture. The end result therefore remains very poor.

Case Z16 (Table 2.2, No. 5): Transtemporal decompression on 9th day of palsy, after complete degeneration had been found on the 7th day (1st day of examination). Further examination not possible for external reasons.

Case Z17 (Table 2.2, No. 7): Degeneration already complete by 1st examination day (8th day of palsy). Transtemporal decompression on 9th day. Beginning of regeneration and function recovery recognizable by 120th day, with clear progress up to 170th day. The outlook for good functional recovery appears favorable, but the risk of an evolution similar to that of Z14 cannot be excluded.

Case Z19 (Table 2.2, No. 9): Patient came for first examination on 15th day of palsy. At that time degeneration was complete. Transtemporal decompression was postponed until the 28th day because of bacterial superinfection of herpes rash in region of outer ear. Satisfactory regeneration and recovery of function in spite of fairly strong associated movement.

Case V3 (Table 2.3, No. 2): The patient presented for the first time on the 18th day of palsy, by which time degeneration had reached 89% and halted. Transtemporal decompression on 33rd day, at a time when the rules for prognosis set out in Section 3.5.0 had not yet been formulated.

3.7. Indications for Transtemporal Decompression of the Facial Nerve

It is not the aim of this work to make a case for or against operative treatment of facial palsy. All that is envisaged is a statement of position. The problem is extremely complex, and many aspects still have to be thoroughly considered. We have already noted in the foreword that in the light of combined clinical and electromyographic investigations we came to the conclusion that decompression of the facial nerve involving the opening of the tympanic or mastoidal section of the fallopian canal is ineffective. The new technique of transtemporal access to the internal auditory canal, developed by House (1961) was first applied by Fisch in an attempt to explore unknown fields in cases of herpes oticus and idiopathic facial palsy. The opening of the internal auditory canal and the adjoining labyrinthine section of the fallopian canal soon revealed why the previous, and now obsolete, approach was useless. The relevant pathogenetic processes were occuring some 1–2 cm further proximally than had been assumed, and therefore could not be observed before. It will be evident to those who seek enlightenment that on the basis of the findings described in the first part of this treatise the site for decompression, if the method is selected, should be only the section of the nerve in the region of the entrance to the facial canal, i.e., decompression should be only transtemporal.

Our investigations have shown that a degree of degeneration of 95% is critical. If more than 95% of the facial motor fibers degenerate, the prognosis becomes doubtful, and if more than 98% degenerate, then only in a small number of patients will recovery of function reach the level of satisfactory to good. One of the conditions governing a decision to operate may therefore be expressed as follows: Transtemporal decompression can only be considered for those patients where a degree of degeneration of 95% or more has been reached, or will be reached.

One extremely difficult problem that arises is to predict in which patients degeneration is likely to reach this critical point, and to do so before the 10th day of palsy, and if at all possible between the 4th and 8th days. This is because degeneration at the point of strangulation reaches its definitive extent by the 10th day at the latest (cf. 3.4.2.1) and yet only becomes detectable by electroneurography on the 11th or 12th day, while the aim of transtemporal decompression is to halt the process before the 95% barrier is reached. It is evident that the electroneurographic method, although the most precise in other contexts, does not suffice for such a purpose. Yet there is no other known method of making more accurate predictions. We must therefore fall back on prognostic methods of the type shown in Table 3.16 (cf. also 3.5.0). From this table it would appear that 95% degeneration or more will be reached if there is at least 40% on the 4th day, 50% on the 5th day, 60% on the 6th day, 70% on the 7th, 80% on the 8th, and 90% on the 9th. With the help of the table the indications for operation can already be weighed between the 4th and 8th days. It is nevertheless unlikely that in observation of these criteria an operation will be carried out on a patient who in fact does not reach the critical point. It is of course quite possible that patients whose readings may lie around the indicated values for some days will go on to reach the critical point. But it is much more important to make sure that an operation is not carried out on a patient who has no need of it, than to interpret the rules too rigidly and operate on all patients who fulfil the time period criteria. It should never be forgotten that this is an intervention more for "cosmetic" than any vital considerations, and that even when degeneration is complete there still remains a chance for a small number of patients to make a satisfactory and spontaneous recovery of function.

Moreover, the indications for operation are subject to further constraints: (1) *Age.* We regard any age over 70 as an aboslute contraindication, and an age over 60 as a relative contraindication. (2) *General condition.* Since this is not a vital operation, the overall risks, including anesthesia, can only be considered acceptable if the patient's general condition is really good. The patient's affectivity must also be considered in this context: depressive and subdepressive patients should be excluded. (3) *Comprehension and adaptation.* It should be clear that transtemporal decompression can only be carried out after the patient has been fully informed of what is involved, and has affirmed a strong desire for it.

It is difficult to make estimates at present regarding the future outlook for the technique of transtemporal decompression of the facial nerve. It presents a number of difficulties: a major one is that it involves an exacting microsurgical intervention, which has to be carried out intracranially and in the immediate vicinity of the brain. Complete mastery of the specialized operating technique is an essential requirement if the risks are to be kept within acceptable limits. If we are to be consistent, it must be possible to carry out the operation as an emergency at weekends. The preoperative diagnostics must also be of a high level. We should like once more to emphasize that the excitability test can no longer be considered as an arguably valid diagnostic basis in the establishment of the indications for transtemporal decompression; still less can gustometry.

A further limiting condition is created by the fact that a considerable number of patients present to the physician for the first time only by the 10th day of palsy or later. If the indications are to be strictly interpreted, then it could be said that the operation is not indicated after the 10th day. However, a plea could be made for a prolongation of the acceptable period for operation, with an eye to conservation of the nerve connective tissue. This is because the outcome for the connective tissue cannot be linked with as much certainty to the 10th day of palsy as it is for the axons. We are of the opinion that in regard to the total extent of damage there is not much difference concerning time elapsed between the nerve fibers and the connective tissue. But naturally it can also be argued that decompression of the strangulated connective tissue even between the 10th and 15th days can still improve the chances of regeneration, which as already frequently emphasized, depend above all on the general condition of the tissue.

As matters stand at present, it cannot be said that we are in possession of unequivocal and fully tested indications for transtemporal decompression. An exception, however, that can be made to this general statement is in relation to those herpes oticus cases where, in addition to facial palsy, there are clear signs of vestibular and cochlear involvement. If decompression is carried out in the early days of palsy onset, even where a high degree of degeneration has not been reached (Z4), the duration of illness can be considerably shortened and the outlook for good functional recovery by the facial muscles is improved. Cases Z4 and Z8 have a certain value as evidence of this, although they could not be considered as providing statistical support, in terms of numbers.

Transtemporal decompression of the facial nerve is at present an intervention that can be fully defended providing that the reservations expressed here are observed. As a result of the technique we have considerably extended our knowledges of the pathogenetically relevant processes in the facial nerve. Even if it is never carried out as a "routine" intervention it still has the merit of having at long last invalidated the use of mastoidal decompression, which is useless for the purpose it was conceived for.

3.8. On Drug Therapy of Idiopathic Facial Palsy

The first communication in regard to the effectiveness of cortisone in the treatment of Bell's palsy appeared in 1951. A number of communications followed, in which in individual cases cortisone treatment was described as having a favourable effect on the course of facial palsy. In the course of time the number of patients available for evaluation continued to increase, and some skeptical voices made themselves heard. Mueller and Mumenthaler (1963) investigated 278 cases and found no difference between prednisolone therapy and conservative methods of treatment. Schliack (1973) also said he was convinced that steroid therapy had no real effect, but Adour et al. (1972) of the

Facial Paralysis Research Clinic in Oakland were much more optimistic. Against this stands the most recent communication from the U. S. (May M., personal communication): "We can now state with statistical support rather than impression that *steroids do not alter the natural history of Bell's palsy.*" Thus, in 23 years of international discussion, no consensus has yet emerged on the simple question of whether steroid therapy is useful or not.

This treatise does not seek to settle the problem—what is aimed at here is rather to prepare the methodology by which questions of this kind can be reliably answered.

A review of the literature to date concerning prednisolone therapy in idiopathic facial palsy shows that very little attention has been paid to the time relationship between the day of palsy onset and the beginning of treatment. If, however, the findings described in Sections 3.4.2 to 3.5.0 are taken as a basis, and we also bear in mind that nerve fiber degeneration is completed by the 10th day of palsy at the latest, it is evident that no pertinent observation can be made about a specific treatment unless particular attention is given to the time point when it begins. The results will be invalidated if patients whose treatment begins, say, after the 5th day of palsy, are mixed with those whose treatment began on the 1st or 2nd day of palsy. Another requirement is that patient groups must be classified strictly in accordance with the day of palsy onset and the day of beginning of treatment, respectively, in order to assess the therapeutic effects. The core group, from which the statistical assessment will be made, should include only those patients whose treatment begins at the latest by the 2nd day of palsy. If the case histories of a sufficiently large group of such patients are taken, and compared with those of an untreated group of the same age, valid assessments can be pronounced. Patients whose treatment begins later can only be included in the evaluation if they are placed in clearly defined groups in regard to the interval day of palsy onset and beginning of treatment (e.g., on 5th and 6th day of palsy, and so on).

The same requirements apply, mutatis mutandis, to the evaluation of transtemporal decompression. But two things must be kept in mind: (1) Only in exceptional cases (Z4, Z8) it is possible to make a decision on the indications before the 4th day of palsy. As a general rule, the signs of an unfavorable course can only be assessed with sufficient reliability between the 6th and 8th days. (2) The inevitable disadvantages of delaying operative therapy are compensated by the considerably more rapid effect: the swollen and strangulated nerve is immediately relieved, and even under the operation microscope the first signs can be seen of drainage of the edema from the released nerve.

Whether or not prednisolone is effective in this particular sense in relieving the facial nerve has not yet been established, but in any case one should allow for an intervening period of at least 2–3 days before the pathogenetically relevant processes have been halted to such an extent that no further nerve fiber degeneration ensues. There is certainly nothing to be gained by continuing steroid therapy beyond the 14th day of palsy.

Summary

1. The transtemporal opening of the internal auditory and the facial channel in patients with acute facial palsies has revealed that the pathogenetically essential processes are localized at the entrance to the fallopian canal. During the acute phase of nerve affection, observation of the facial nerve with the operation microscope regularly shows an enormous edema with considerable hemorrhagic infarction of the nerve before entering the facial canal, and heavy strangulation at the transition from the relatively wide fundus of the internal auditory canal to the facial canal.

On intratemporal stimulation of the facial nerve a conduction block can be localized in the nerve segment immediately inside the entrance to the facial canal. *There is complete correspondence between the morphologic and functional alteration of nerve.*

The prevailing concept of the localization of nerve damage in the distal segments of the facial canal has to be abandoned. The changes occasionally to be observed in the tympanic and mastoidal segment are nothing but remote signs of the decisive processes taking place at the entrance to the fallopian canal. It is not surprising that there is a certain spreading of these changes to more distal parts of the nerve, but this does not mean that this is the main site of nerve affection as has hitherto been assumed. Therefore, decompression of the facial nerve can be worthwhile–but only at the entrance to the fallopian canal. Decompression of facial nerve in the segments distal to chorda tympani is an obsolete intervention of proved ineffectiveness.

2. The rather uniform morphologic aspect in all cases of acute facial palsy of different etiologies suggests a strongly determining influence of "local" factors on the sequence of pathogenetic events. Decisive for the degree of nerve damage are obviously not the different etiologic factors but the intensity of the local processes triggered by them. The congruence of the essential pathogenetic features in acute facial palsies of different etiology was until now unknown. The doctrine of initial vasospasm and primary ischemia in idiopathic facial palsy has not been proven and is superfluous. Considerations on pathogenesis must include the importance of intraneural microcirculation based on experimental work.

3. The congruence in the pathogenesis of facial palsies of different etiologies justifies the summarizing denomination "acute facial palsies". In order to distinguish these from the palsies caused by bacterial infections of the middle ear which are nowadays rare, one can specify them as acute, nonbacterial facial palsies or include the localization: acute meatolabyrinthine facial palsies, or acute facial palsies of meatolabyrinthine localization.

4. A modification of the electroneurographic method allows the indication of the degree of degeneration of the paretic facial nerve directly in percent.

5. The processes causing degeneration in acute facial palsies spontaneously come to an end no later than the 10th day of palsy.

6. In idiopathic facial palsy loss of innervation of facial muscles is generally due partly to nerve fiber degeneration and partly to blocked impulse conduction. Only 4 out of 145 cases (2.75%) showed no signs of degeneration whatsoever and only 9 (6.20%) degeneration of all motor fibers.

7. The duration of the conduction block is correlated to the degree of degeneration: the higher the percentage of degenerated fibers the longer the delay until recovery of blocked fibers.

8. Latency between nerve stimulation and muscle action potential statistically increases with higher degrees of degeneration. In the individual case, however, latency is not a useful parameter for evaluation of prognosis.

9. Up to a degree of 50% degeneration, functional recovery is always very good. Time required for recovery is generally between 6 and 7 weeks.

10. Up to a degree of 90% degeneration, recovery is nearly always very good and only few cases show some inconspicuous signs of permanent paralysis. In contrast to patients with degeneration of up to 50% the time course of recovery is considerably longer (up to 3 times as long).

11. Up to 98% of degeneration, most patients reach a satisfying degree of functional recovery. In fact, for some, recovery may be excellent. Only few cases show poor recovery, frequently in connection with misdirection of regenerating axons (associated movements) manifesting itself for the first time in this range of degeneration.

12. With 98–100% degeneration, recovery is unsatisfactory or poor in most patients. In exceptional cases good recovery can occur even with this high degree of degeneration.

13. Most patients with poor recovery show associated movements as sequelae of misdirection of regenerating axons. This misdirection is a consequence of the destruction of endoneurial tubes and of formation of intraneural scars by damaged connective tissue. The degree of damage to intraneural connective tissue is of decisive importance for recovery of nerve function.

14. In young patients, recovery is statistically quicker and better than in old ones. Even in young patients, however, nerve degeneration may be complete.

15. Degeneration up to 50% is clinically unrecognizable as long as impulse conduction of the remaining 50% of fibers is not disturbed.

16. The above-quoted rules are valid for all acute facial palsies. This statement does not exclude the fact that certain etiologies tend to more severe courses than others. Facial palsy with herpes oticus is on the average related to higher degrees of degeneration than Bell's palsy.

17. Bilateral facial palsies occurring with lymphocytic meningitis and polyradiculitis show a remarkable parallelism of the course of degeneration and regeneration of both nerves. This suggests an early determination of the whole course.

18. The electroneurographic method described allows reliable prognosis not later than on the 10th day of palsy, in many cases 2–3 days earlier. The trend to an unfavorable course can be detected much earlier than hitherto.

19. The transtemporal decompression of the facial nerve is still in a phase of examination. It seems likely to be very useful in cases of peracute herpes zoster oticus on the 2nd to 4th day if there is involvement of the vestibular and/or cochlear nerve.

20. The very short duration of the acute phase of facial palsies implies that valid statements on the effectiveness of drug (steroid) therapy can be made only on the bases of strictly homogenous groups of patients with respect to the time relation between the beginning of therapy to the onset of palsy. One should insist that statistical statements be based on observation of a sufficiently large number of patients where therapy is started not later than the day after onset of palsy.

References

Aboulker, P., Cathala, H. P., Demaldent, J. E., Chouard, C. H.: Réinnervation par les nerfs voisins. Evolution électromyographique d'une paralysie faciale traumatique. J. franç. Oto-rhinolaryng. **16**, 277–279 (1967)

Adour, K. K., Swanson, P. J.: Facial paralysis in 403 consecutive patients: emphasis on treatment response in patients with Bell's palsy. Trans. Amer. Acad. Ophthal. Otolaryng. **75**, 1284–1301 (1971)

Adour, K. K., Wingerd, J., Bell, D. N., Manning, J. J., Hurley, J. P.: Prednisolone treatment for idiopathic facial paralysis (Bell's palsy). New Engl. J. Med. **287**, 1268–1272 (1972)

Alexander, G.: Zur Klinik und pathologischen Anatomie der sog. „rheumatischen" Facialislähmung. Arch. Psychiat. **35**, 778–786 (1902)

Alford, B. R., Weber, S. C., Sessions, R. B.: Neurodiagnostic studies in facial paralysis. Ann. Otol. (St. Louis) **79**, 227–233 (1970)

Altman, A. J.: Facial nucleus in Bell's palsy. Bull. Johns Hopk. Hosp. **118**, 265–274 (1966)

André-Thomas: Contribution à l'étude de l'anatomie pathologique de la paralysie faciale périphérique et de l'hémispasme faciale (Trois cas suivis d'autopsie). Rev. neurol. **15**, 1273–1277 (1907)

Baker, A. B.: Disorders of the brain stem and its cranial nerves. In: Clinical Neurology, 2nd Ed. New York (1962)

Bethlem, J.: Herpetic geniculate ganglionitis. Acta neuropath. (Berl.) **2**, 97–101 (1962)

Blackley, B., Friedmann, J., Wright, I.: Herpes Zoster auris associated with facial nerve palsy and auditory nerve symptoms. Acta oto-laryng. (Stockh.) **63**, 533–550 (1967)

Blinkov, S. M., Glezer, I. I.: Das Zentralnervensystem in Zahlen und Tabellen. Jena: VEB Gustav Fischer 1968

Blunt, M. J.: Ischemic degeneration of nerve fibers. Arch. Neurol. (Chic.) **2**, 528–536 (1960).

Blunt, M. J.: The possible role of vascular changes in the aetiology of Bell's palsy. J. Laryng. **70**, 701–713 (1956)

Blunt, M. J.: The blood supply of the facial nerve. J. Anat. (Lond.) **88**, 520–526 (1954)

Bobby, R.: Electrodiagnostic studies in facial paralysis. Arch. Otolaryng. (Chic.) **85**, 259–264 (1967)

Boyle, W. F.: Facial-nerve paralysis: An experimental investigation of facial nerve regeneration in monkeys. Laryngoscope (St. Louis) **76**, 1921–1948 (1966)

Boyle, W. F.: Evaluation of facial nerve decompression in experimental facial nerve paralysis in monkeys. Laryngoscope (St. Louis) **77**, 1168–1178 (1967)

Buchthal, F.: Electromyography in paralysis of the facial nerve. Arch. Otolaryng. **81**, 463–469 (1965)

Buskirk, C., van: The seventh nerve complex. J. comp. Neurol. **82**, 303–333 (1945)

Cathala, H.-P., Chouard, C.-H., Pierrot-Deseilligny, E.: Pathogénie de la dissociation de la paralysie centrale. Argument nouveau d'ordre électromyographique. Ann. Otolaryng. (Paris) **86**, 625–630 (1969)

Cawthorne, T.: Role of surgery in investigation and treatment of peripheral facial palsy. Lancet **1952 I**, 1219–1220

Cawthorne, T.: Peripheral facial paralysis. Some aspects of its pathology. Laryngoscope (St. Louis) **56**, 653–664 (1946)

Chouard, C.-H.: La neurolyse chordale: Nouveau traitement de la paralysie faciale a frigore. Ann. Oto-laryng. (Paris) **87**, 455–464 (1970)

Chouard, C.-H., Charachon, R., Morgon, A., Cathala, H. P.: Anatomie, pathologie et chirurgie du nerf facial. Paris: 1972

Chouard, C.-H., Poulain, H., Mauvais-Jarvis, A.: Localisation dans le tronc du nerf des fibres du territoire facial supérieur. Ann. Oto-laryng. (Paris) **86**, 643–646 (1969)

Coassolo, M.: Ricerche sperimentali sulla paralisi "a frigore" del facciale. Minerva otorinolaring. **2**, 444–449 (1952)

Coassolo, M.: Studio della eccitabilità elettrica del nervo facciale nella paralisi "a frigore" sperimentale. Minerva otorinolaring. **3**, 31–34 (1953)

Coassolo, M.: Azione della novocaina nella paralisi "a frigore" del facciale; ricerche sperimentali. Minerva otorinolaring. **3**, 281–282 (1953)

Darkschewitsch, L., Tichonow, S.: Zur Frage von den pathologisch-anatomischen Veränderungen bei peripherer Facialislähmung nichtspezifischen Ursprungs. Neurol. Cbl. **12**, 329–339 (1893)
Dejerine, J., Theohari, A.: Un cas de paralysis faciale périphérique dite rhumatismale ou "a frigore", suivi d'autopsie. Compt. R. Soc. Biol. (Paris) **49**, 1033–1035 (1897)
Denny-Brown, D., Adams, R. D., Fitzgerald, P. J.: Pathologic features of herpes zoster. Arch. Neurol. Psychiat. (Chic.) **51**, 216–231 (1944)
Denny-Brown, D., Brenner, C.: Paralysis of nerve induced by direct pressure and by tourniquet. Arch. Neurol. Psychiat. (Chic.) **51**, 1–26 (1944a)
Denny-Brown, D., Brenner, C.: Lesion in peripheral nerve resulting from compression by spring clip. Arch. Neurol. Psychiat. **52**, 1–19 (1944b)
Devriese, P. P.: Experiments on the facial nerve. Amsterdam, London: North Holland Publ. 1972
Devriese, P. P.: Facial paralysis in cephalic herpes zoster. Ann. Otol. (St. Louis) **77**, 1101–1119 (1968)
Doboti, M.: Frühjahrsvers. Schweizer ORL-Ges., Neuchâtel, 1973
Esslen, E.: Electromyographic findings on two types of misdirection of regenerating axions. J. EEG Clin. Neurophysiol. **12**, 738–741 (1959)
Esslen, E.: Electromyographic findings on two types of misdirection of regenerating axons. J. electroenceph. clin. Neurophysiol. **12**, 738–741 (1960)
Esslen, E.: Electrodiagnosis of facial palsy. In: Miehlke, A.: Surgery of the Facial Nerve. Munich, London, Toronto: Urban und Schwarzenberg, 1973
Esslen, E., Fisch, U.: Zur Lokalisation der Nervenschädigung bei der idiopathischen Facialisparese und zur Frage der Dekompression. Schweiz. med. Wschr. **101**, 386–387 (1971)
Eyriès, Ch., Chouard, C.-H.: Le faisceau solitaire et ses noyaux. Ann. Oto-laryng. (Paris) **82**, 15–36 (1965)
Eyriès, Ch., Chouard, C.-H.: Les voies cochléaires bulbo-protubérantielles. Problèmes Actuels d'O. R. L. 1970
Eyriès, Ch., Chouard, C.-H.: Les origines réelles du nerf facial. Ann. Oto-laryng. (Paris) **80**, 775–802 (1963)
Findlay, J. P.: Facial paralysis: a clinical review with an autopsy report of the histopathology in a case of infection of the geniculate ganglion by the virus of cephalic herpes zoster. Med. J. Aust. **2**, 810–812 (1952)
Fisch, U.: The surgical anatomy of the so-called internal auditory atery. Nobel Symp. 10: Disorders of the Skull Base Region, Stockholm 1968
Fisch, U.: Transtemporal surgery of the internal auditory canal. Advanc. Oto-rino-laryng. **17**, 203–240 (1970)
Fisch, U. : In: A. Miehlke: Surgery of the Facial Nerve. Munich, Philadelphia: Urban und Schwarzenberg 1973
Fisch, U.: Proc. 3rd Int. Symp. on Facial Nerve Surgery, Zurich, Aug. 9–12, 1976 (in press)
Fisch, U., Esslen, E.: Total intratemporal exposure of the facial nerve. Arch. Otolaryng. **95**, 335–341 (1972)
Fisch, U., Esslen, E.: Zur chirurgischen Behandlung der idiopathischen Facialisparese. Méd. et Hyg. (Geneva) **28**, 1591–1592 (1970)
Fisch, U., Esslen, E.: Zur Frage der Re-Innervation der Gesichtsmuskulatur nach Resektion des zugehörigen N. facialis. Pract. Oto-rhino-laryng. (Basle) **30**, 1–13 (1968)
Foley, J. O.: The special visceral efferent zone of the seventh cranial nerve in the canalis facialis. J. comp. Neurol. **88**, 439–451 (1948)
Fowler, E. P., jr.: The pathologic findings in a case of facial paralysis. Trans. Amer. Acad. Ophthal. Otolaryng. **67** (1963)
Fowler, T. J., Danta, G., Gilliatt, R. W.: Recovery of nerve conduction after a pneumatic tourniquet: observations on the hind-limb of the baboon. J. Neurol. Neurosurg. Psychiat. **35**, 638–647 (1972)
Fox, J. L., Kenmore, P. I.: The effect of ischemia on nerve conduction. Exp. Neurol. **17**, 403–419 (1967)
Glasscock, M. E. III, House, W. F., Alford, B. R.: Middle fossa facial nerve decompression. Ann. Otol. (St. Louis) **79**, 234–240 (1970)
Grose, C., Henle, W., Henle, G. et al.: Primary Epstein-Barr-virus infections in acute neurological diseases. New Engl. J. Med. **202**, 392–395 (1975)

Grünberg, H.: Zur Histopathologie des Zoster oticus. Arch. Ohr., Nas.- u. Kehlk.-Heilk. **177**, 187–192 (1961)
Guerrier, Y.: In: Proc. 3rd Int. Symp. on Facial Nerve Surgery, Fisch, U. (ed.), Zurich, Aug. 9–12, 1976
Guldberg-Möller, J., Olsen, S., Kettel, K.: Histopathology of the facial nerve in herpes zoster oticus. Arch. Otolaryng. **69**, 266–275 (1959)
Gutmann, E.: Die funktionelle Regeneration der peripheren Nerven. Berlin: Akademie-Verlag, 1958
Hall, A.: Pathology of Bell's palsy. Arch. Otolaryng. **54**, 475–477 (1951).
Heilborn, F.: Morphologische Studien zur Pathogenese des Zoster. Acta anat. (Basle) **10**, 363–376 (1950)
Hilger, J. A.: The nature of Bell's palsy. Laryngoscope (St. Louis) **59**, 228–235 (1949)
Hofmann, C.: Der Faserverlauf im N. facialis. Z. Hals-, Nas.- u. Ohrenheilk. **10**, 86 (1924)
House, W. F.: Surgical exposure of the internal auditory canal and its contents through the middle cranial fossa. Laryngoscope **71**, 1363–1385 (1961)
Hunt, J. R.: On herpetic inflammation of the geniculate ganglion. A new syndrome and its complications. J. nerv. ment. Dis. **34**, 73 (1907)
James, J.: Einige Bemerkungen über die Histologie des Nervus facialis zur Pathogenese der Bell'schen Lähmung. Z. Laryng. Rhinol. **40**, 336–337 (1961)
Jepsen, O.: Topognosis (topographic diagnosis) of facial nerve lesions. Arch. Otolaryng. **81**, 446–456 (1965)
Jongkees, L. B. W.: On the histology of Bell's palsy. Acta otolaryng. (Stockh.) **44**, 336–343 (1954)
Jongkees, L. B. W.: Treatment of Bell's palsy. Neurology (Minneap.) **7**, 697–702 (1957)
Jongkees, L. B. W.: The timing of surgery in intra-temporal facial paralysis. Laryngoscope (St. Louis) **79**, 1557–1561 (1969)
Kaeser, H. E., Pfaltz, C. R.: Elektromyographische Verlaufsuntersuchungen bei Facialisparesen. Confin. neurol. (Basle) **23**, 256–269 (1963)
Kettel, K.: Bell's palsy. Pathology and surgery. Arch. Otolaryng. **46**, 427–472 (1947)
Kettel, K.: Peripheral Facial Palsy. Copenhagen: Munksgaard 1959
Köster, G.: Klinischer und experimenteller Beitrag zur Lehre von der Lähmung des Nervus facialis, zugleich Beitrag zur Physiologie des Geschmackes, der Schweiß-, Speichel- und Thränenabsonderung. Dtsch. Arch. klin. Med. **68**, 343–382 (1900)
Kullman, G. L., Dijck, P. J., Cody, D. T. R.: Anatomy of the mastoid portion of the facial nerve. Arch. Otolaryng. **93**, 29–33 (1971)
Lämmli, K., Fisch, U.: Vestibular symptoms in idiopathic facial palsy. Acta oto-laryng. (Stockh.) **78**, 15–18 (1974)
Larens, W.: Über Schmerzen bei der peripheren Facialislähmung. Nervenarzt **26**, 111–114 (1955)
Laumans, E. P. J.: Nerve excitability tests in facial paralysis. Arch. Otolaryng. **81**, 478–485 (1965)
Lindeman, H.: The Fallopian canal. Acta oto-laryng. (Stockh.) **158**, 204–211 (1960)
Lundborg, G.: Ischemic nerve injury. Scand. J. Plastic reconstr. Surg. Suppl. 6, Stockholm 1970
Mathog, R. H., Mudson, W. R.: Electrodiagnosis in facial palsy. Sth. med. J. (Bgham, Ala.) **63**, 37–40 (1970).
May, M.: Facial paralysis peripheral type: a proposed method of reporting. Laryngoscope (St. Louis) **80**, 331–390 (1970)
May, M.: In: Proc. 3rd Int. Symp. on Facial Nerve surgery, Fisch, U. (ed.). Zurich, Aug. 9–12, 1976 (in press)
Maybaum, J. L., Druss, J. G.: Geniculate ganglionitis (Hunt's syndrome): clinical features and histopathology. Arch. Otolaryng. (Chicago) **19**, 574–581 (1934)
Meyer, A.: Anatomical findings in a case of facial paralysis of ten days duration in a general paralytic, with remarks on the termination of the "auditory" nerves. J. exp. Med. **2**, 607–610 (1897)
Miehlke, A.: Über die Topographie des Faserverlaufs im Facialisstamm. Arch. Ohr.-, Nas.- u. Kehlk.-Heilk. **171**, 340 (1958)
Miehlke, A.: Die ischämische Facialislähmung aus der Sicht des Otochirurgen. Fortschr. Neurol. Psychiat. **27**, 33 (1959)
Miehlke, A.: Die Chirurgie des Nervus facialis. Munich, Berlin 1960
Miehlke, A.: Surgery of the facial nerve, 2nd ed. Munich 1973

Miehlke, A.: Anatomy and clinical aspects of the facial nerve. Arch. Otolaryng. **81**, 444–445 (1965)

Mills, Ch. K.: The sensory functions attributed to the seventh nerve. J. nerv. ment. Dis. **17**, 273–284 (1910).

Minkowski, P.: Zur pathologischen Anatomie der rheumatischen Facialislähmung. Berl. klin. Wschr. **27**, 665–666 (1891)

Mirallié, Ch.: Paralysie faciale périphérique: Autopsie. Rev. neurol. **14**, 792–793 (1906)

Mitrinowicz-Modrzejewska, A.: Vestibular-Chronaxie und ihre Bedeutung für die Untersuchung des taubstimmen Kindes. Arch. Ohr.-, Nas.- u. Kehlk.-Heilk. **172**, 175–179 (1957)

Müller, G., Mumenthaler, M.: Die kryptogenetische Facialisparese. Dtsch. med. Wschr. **88**, 1545–1550 (1963)

Nager, G. T., Nager, M.: The arteries of the human middle ear, with particular regard to the blood of the auditory ossicles. Ann. Otol. (St. Louis) **62**, 923–949 (1953)

Naumann, W. H., Schliack, H., Stüwe, J: Indikation zur Facialisdekompression. Dtsch. med. Wschr. **93**, 1308–1314 (1968)

Ochoa, J., Fowler, T. J., Gilliatt, R. W.: Changes produced by a pneumatic tourniquet. In: New Develop. in Electromyography and Clinic Neurophys. (Ed. J. E. Desmedt) Vol. **2**, p. 174–180. (Karger, Basle: Karger 1973)

Peitersen, E., Andersen, P.: Spontaneous course of 220 peripheral non-traumatic facial palsies. Arch. oto-laryng. (Stockh.) Supp. **224**, 296–300 (1967)

Platau, E.: Pathologisch-anatomischer Befund bei einem Fall peripherer Facialislähmung. Neurolog. Centralbl. **15**, 718–719 (1896)

Proctor, B., Corgill, D. A., Proud, G.: The pathology of Bell's Palsy. Trans. Amer. Acad. Ophthal. Otolaryng. Sect ORL **82**, 70–80 (1976)

Ray, J.: Particularités de l'anatomie du nerf facial chez le nouveau-né. Ann. Oto-laryng. (Paris) **87**, 92–93 (1970)

Rhoton, A. L., O'Leary, J. L., Ferguson, J. P.: The trigeminal, facial, vagal and glossopharyngeal nerves in the monkey. Arch. Neurol. (Chic.) **14**, 530–540 (1966)

Robert, F., Pfaltz, C. R.: Vestibuläre Funktionsstörungen bei idiopathischer Facialisparese (Lokalisations- und Kompensationsprobleme). Arch. Ohr.-, Nas-, u. Kehlk.-Heilk. **197**, 183–192 (1970)

Rosenfalck, P.: Volume conducted action potentials and their correlation to the intracellular potentials. Acta physiol. scand. **42** suppl. **145**, 118–119 (1957)

Sachs, E., House, R. K.: The Ramsay Hunt Syndrome geniculate nerves. Neurology (Minneap.) **6**, 262–268 (1956)

Sachs, E., Jr. Reginald, K.: The Ramsay Hunt syndrome. Geniculate herpes. Neurology (Minneap.) **6**, 262–268 (1956)

Sade, J., Levy, E., Chaco, J.: Surgery and pathology of Bell's palsy. Arch. Otolaryng. (Chicago) **82**, 594–602 (1966)

Schimert, J.: Der Nervus intermedius und das Ganglion geniculi nervi facialis. Zs. mikr.-anat. Forsch. **39**, 1936

Schliack, H.: Zur Therapie der idiopathischen Facialislähmung. Dtsch. Ärztebl. **9**, 562–565 (1973)

Skorpil, W.: The relationship between loss of susceptibility to indirect muscle stimulation and the appearence of denervation fibrillation after section of the facial nerve. Cs. Neurol. **26**, 307–310 (1963)

Steidl, L.: Prognosis and course of Bell's palsy. 1. Clinical study. Arch. Psychiat. Nervenkr. **216**, 311–322 (1972). 2. Electromyographic study. Arch. Psychiat. Nervenkr. **216**, 323–341 (1972)

Sullivan, J. A., Smith, J. B.: The otological concept of Bell's palsy and its treatment. Ann. Otol (St. Louis) **59**, 1142–1170 (1950)

Sunderland, S.: Blood supply of the nerves of the upper limb in man. Arch. Neurol. Psychiat. (Chic.) **53**, 91 (1945a)

Sunderland, S.: Blood supply of peripheral nerves. Practical considerations. Arch. Neurol. Psychiat. (Chic.) **54**, 250 (1945b)

Sunderland, S.: A classification of peripheral nerve injuries producing loss of function. Brain **74**, 491 (1951)

Sunderland, S., Cossar, D. F.: The structure of the facial nerve. Anat. Rec. **116**, 147–165 (1953)

Sunderland, S.: The connective tissues of peripheral nerves. Brain **88**, 841 (1965)

Sunderland, S.: Nerve and nerve injuries. Edinburgh, London: Livingstone 1968

Taverner, D.: Electrodiagnosis in facial palsy. Arch. Otolaryng. **81**, 470–477 (1965)
Tomasch, J.: Über Zahl und Größe der Zellen in den motorischen Hirnnervenkernen des Menschen. Zschr. mikr.-anat. Forsch. **70**, 298–313 (1963)
Tschiassny, K.: Eight syndroms of facial paralysis and their significance in locating lesions. Ann. Otol (St. Louis) **62**, 677–691 (1953)
Wigand, M. E., Spreng, K., Bumm, P.: Auswertungen des Facialis-Elektromyogramms mit dem automatischen Rechner. Archiv Ohr.-, Nas.- u. Kehlk.-Heilk. **191**, 614 (1968a)
Wigand, M. E., Spring, M., Bumm, P.: Computer-Analyse von Facialis-Elektromyogrammen. I. Dauer der Aktionspotentiale. Acta oto-laryng. (Stockh.) **66**, 296–304 (1968b)
Zülch, K. J.: Idiopathic facial paresis. In: Handbook of clinical neurology, Vol. **8**, Amsterdam: North Holland Publ. 1970, p. 241–302

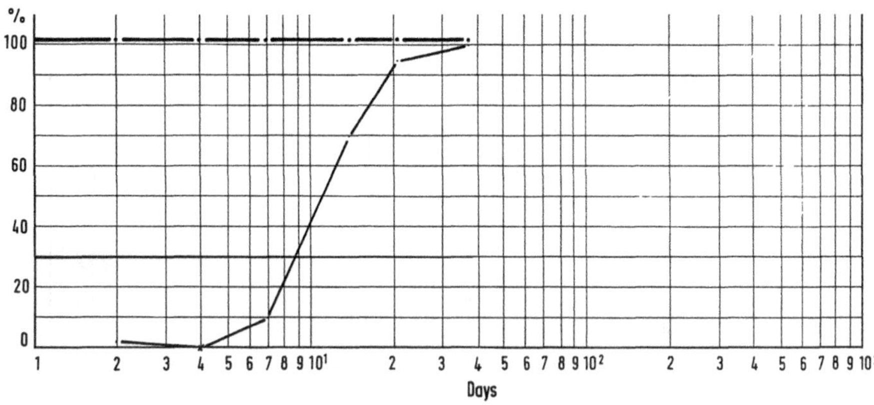

Case 1

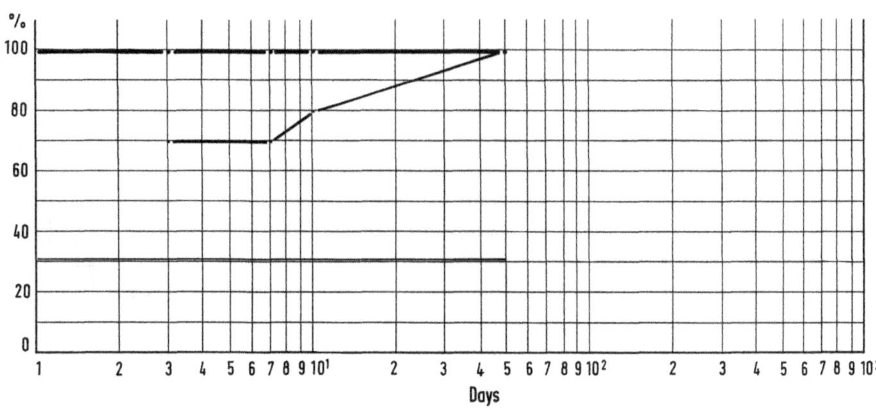

Case 2

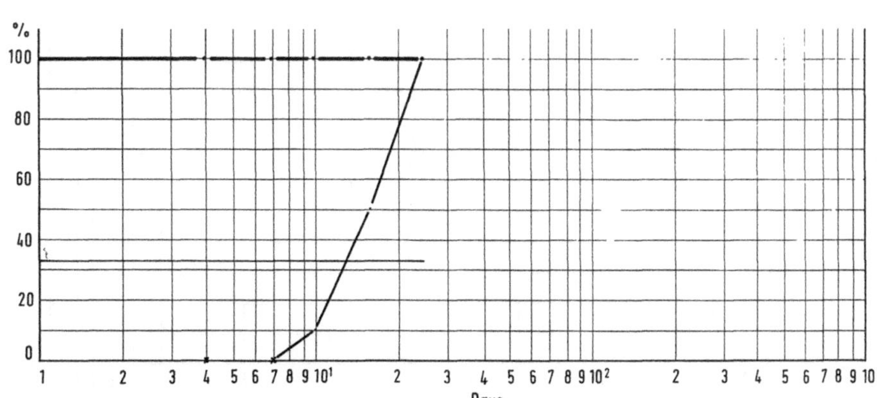

Case 3

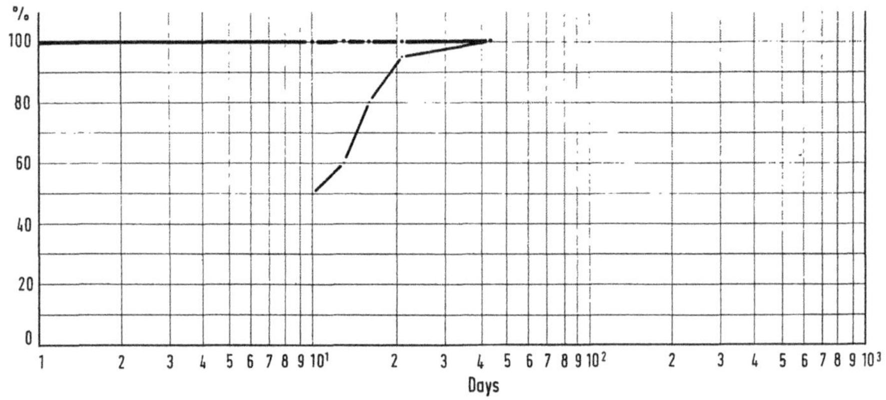

Case 4

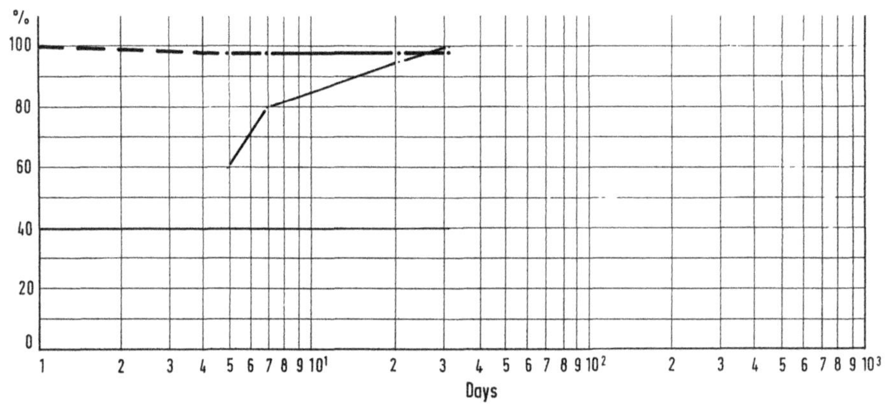

Case 5

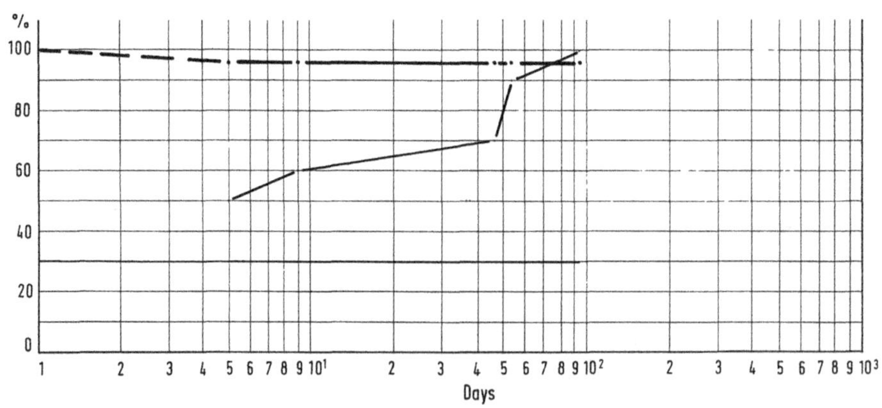

Case 6

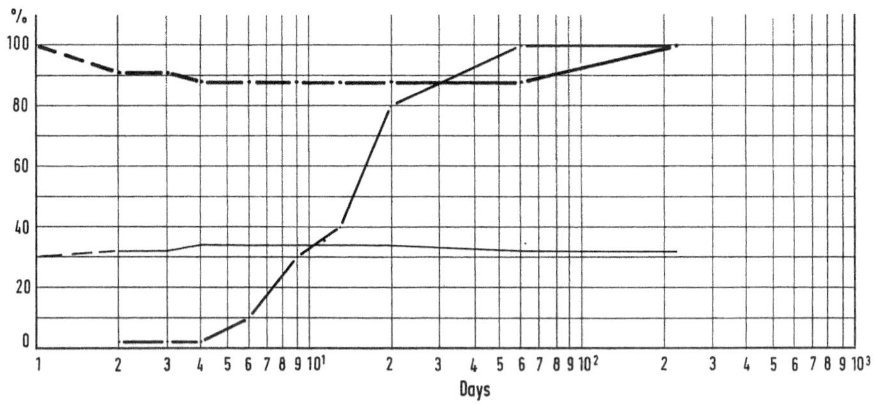

Case 7

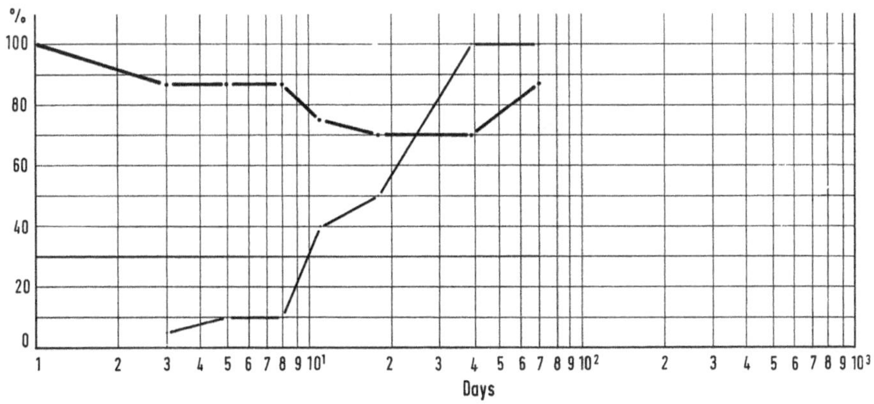

Case 8

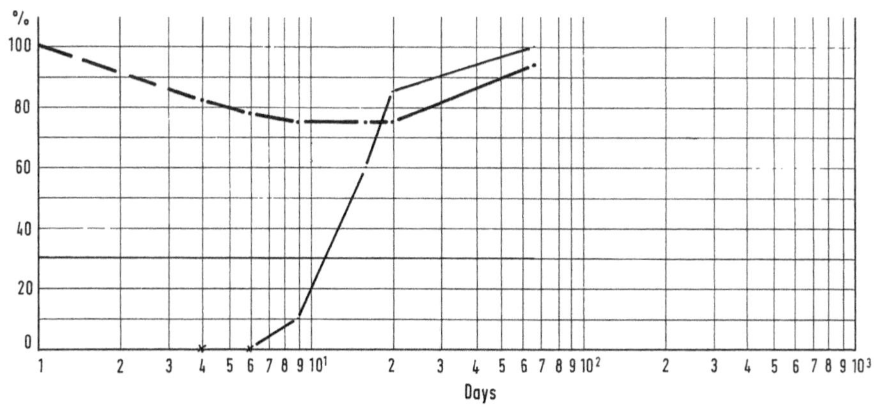

Case 9

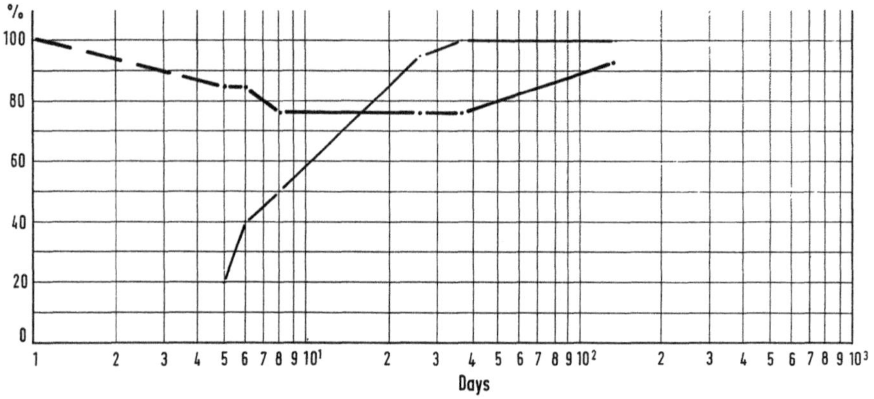

Case 10

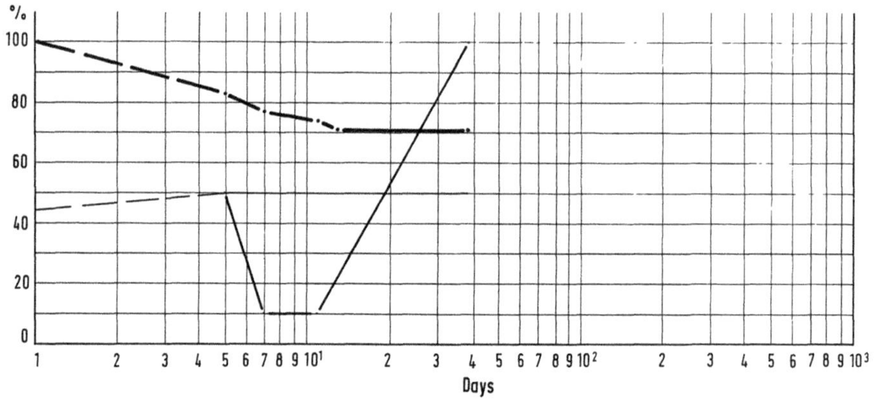

Case 11

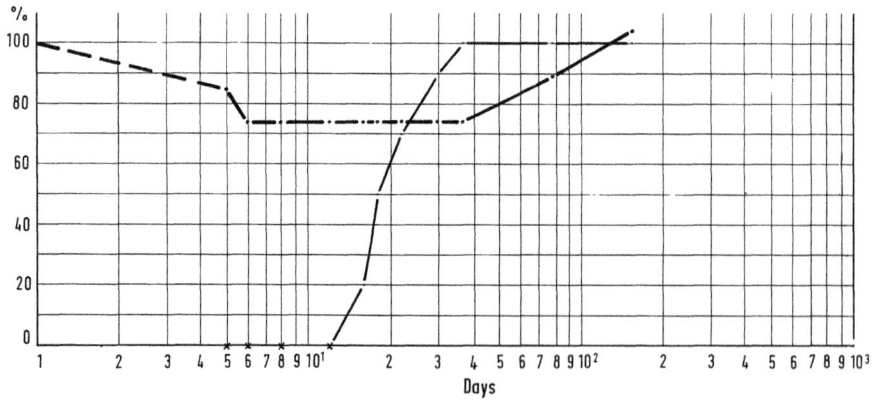

Case 12

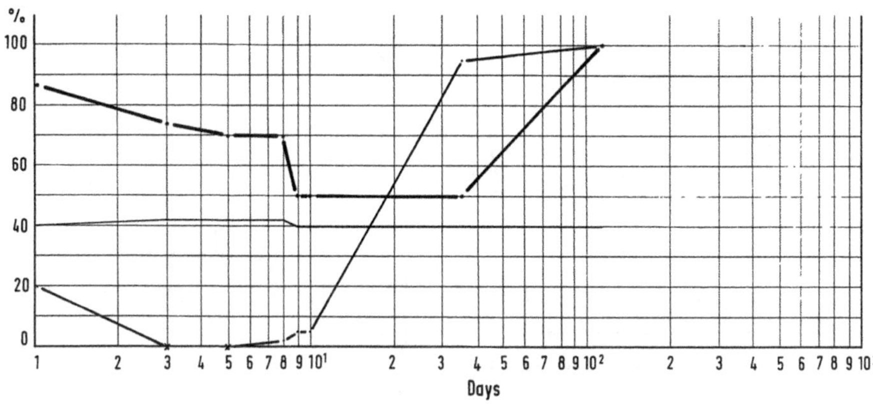

Case 16

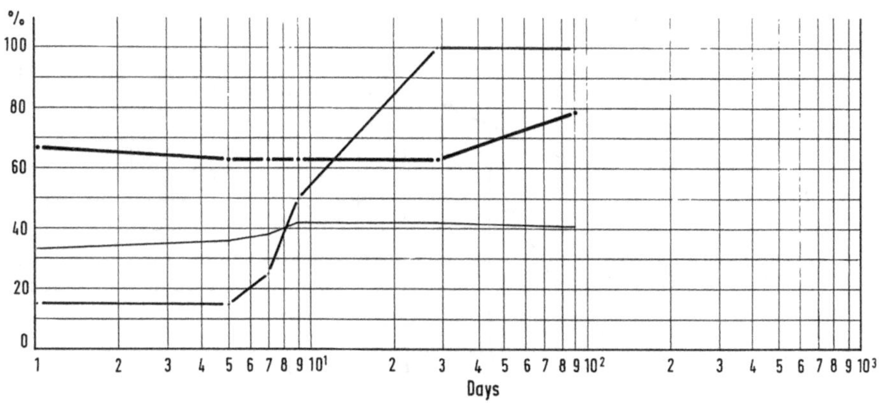

Case 17

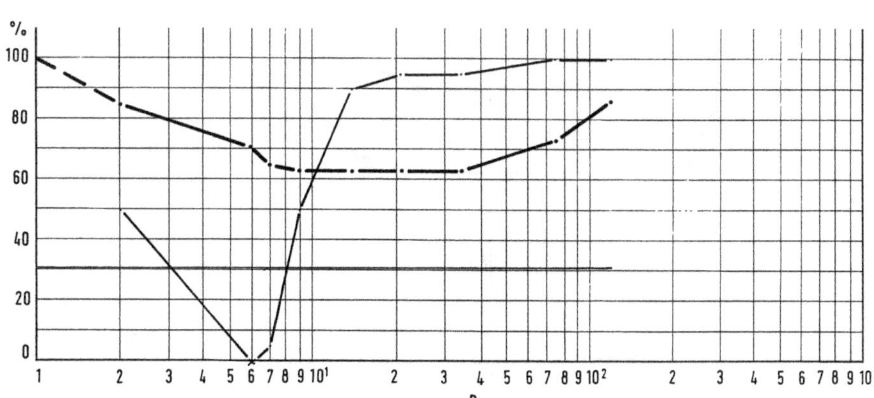

Case 18

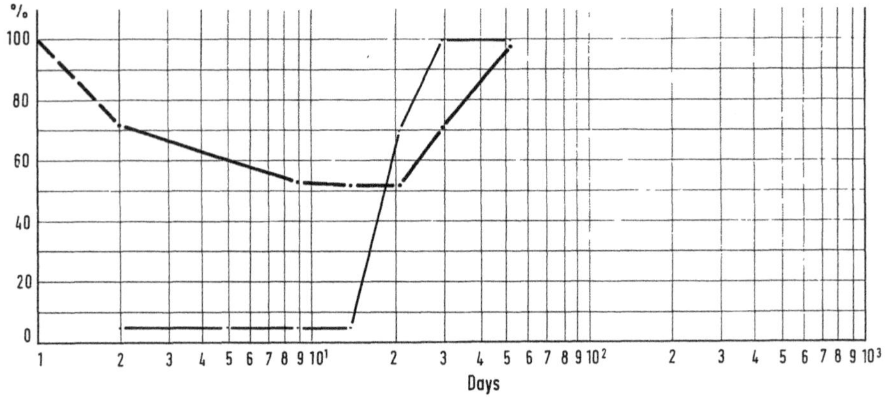

Case 19

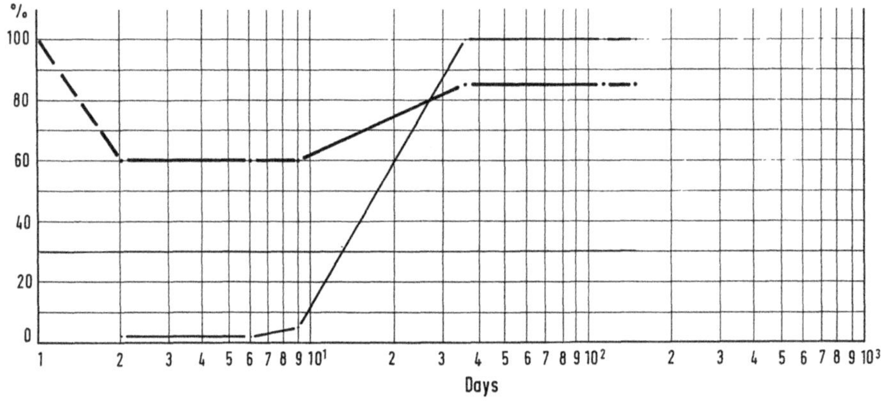

Case 20

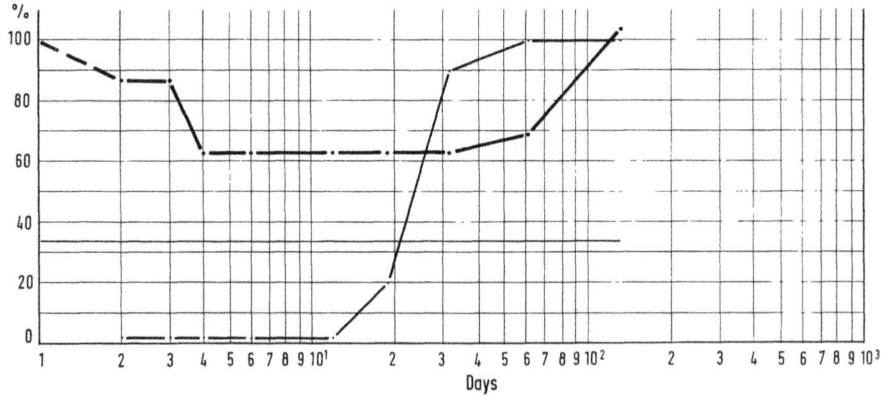

Case 21

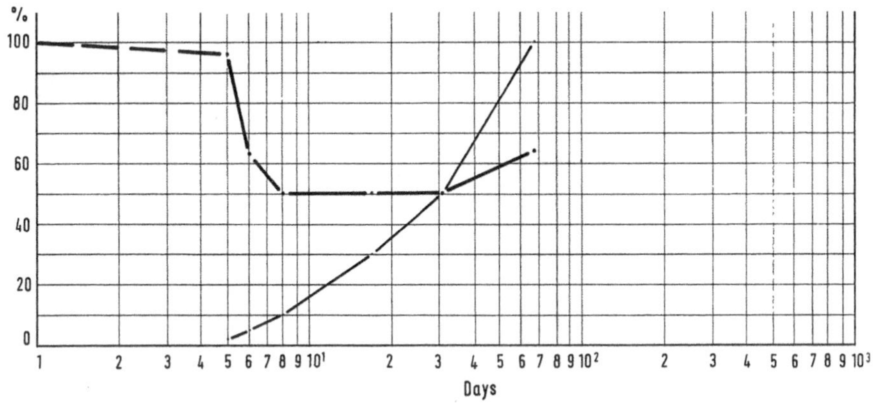

Case 29

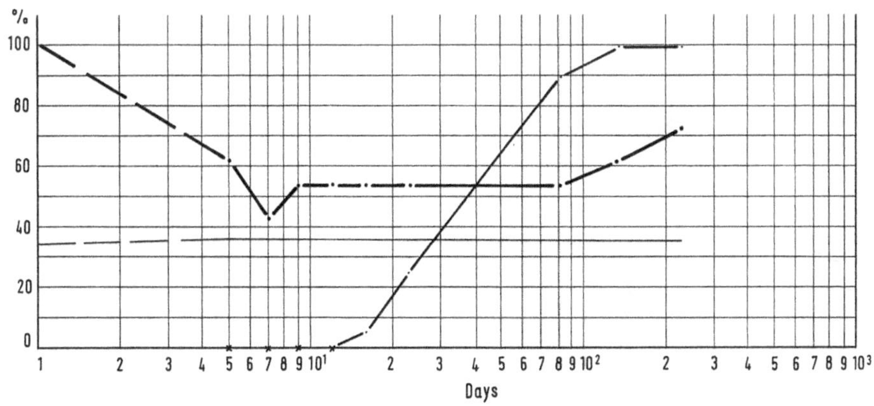

Case 34

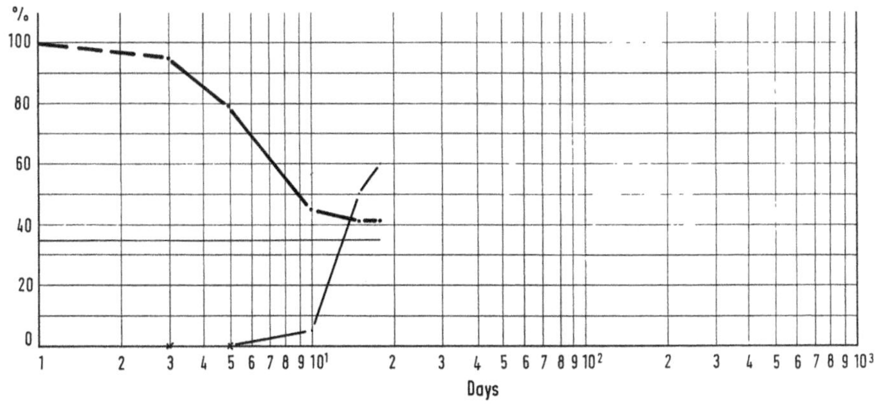

Case 46

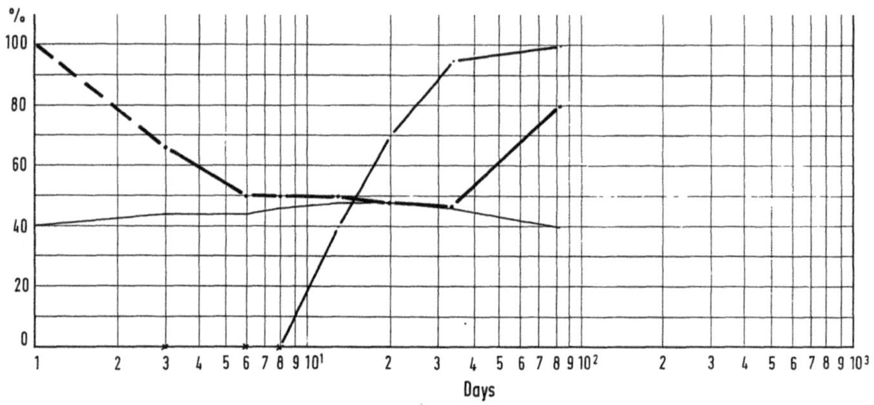

Case 47

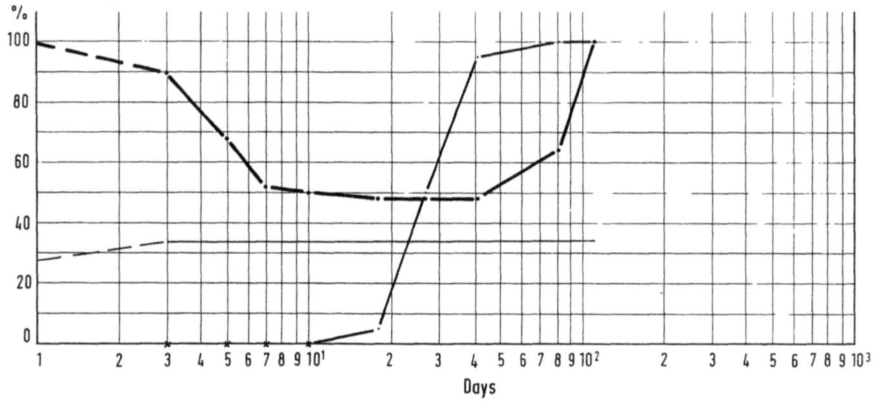

Case 48

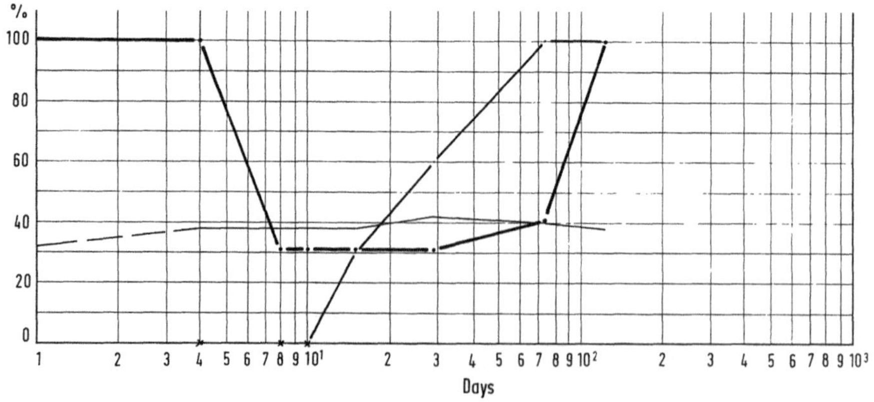

Case 49

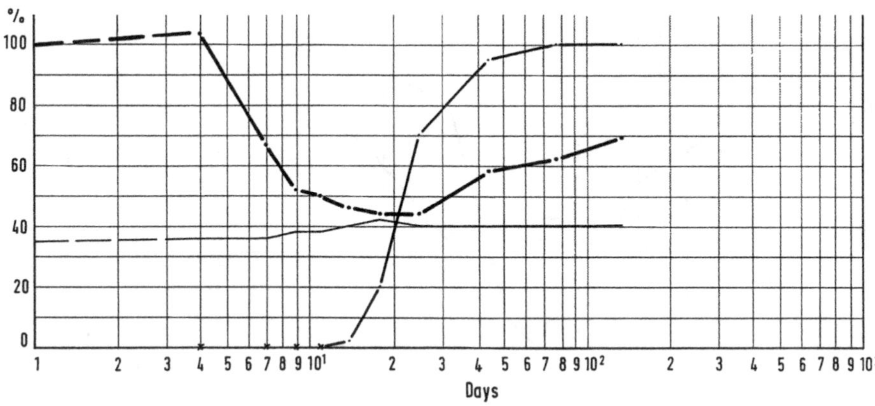

Case 50

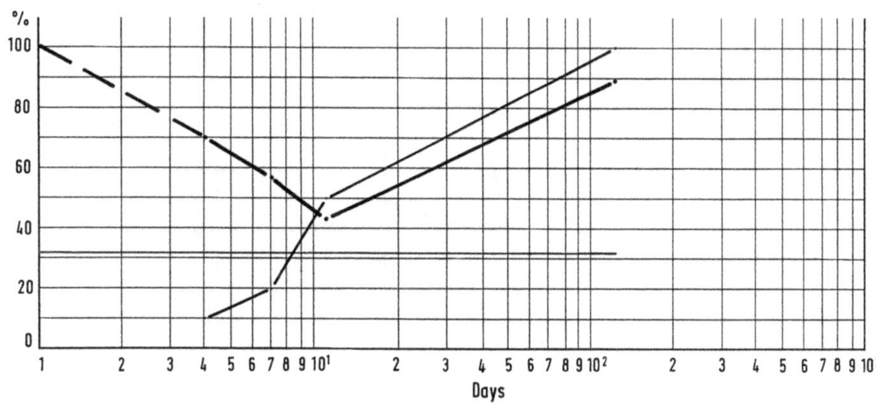

Case 51

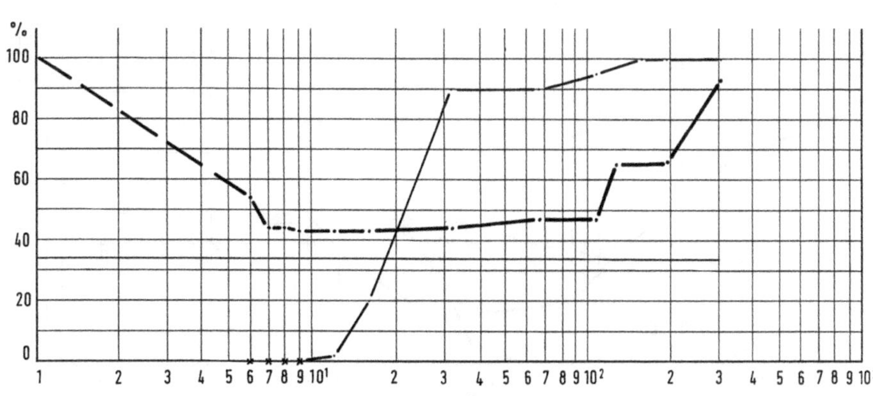

Case 56

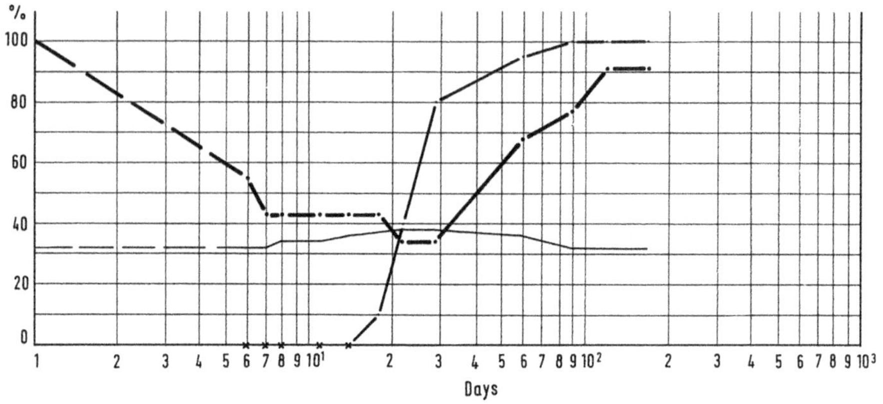

Case 57

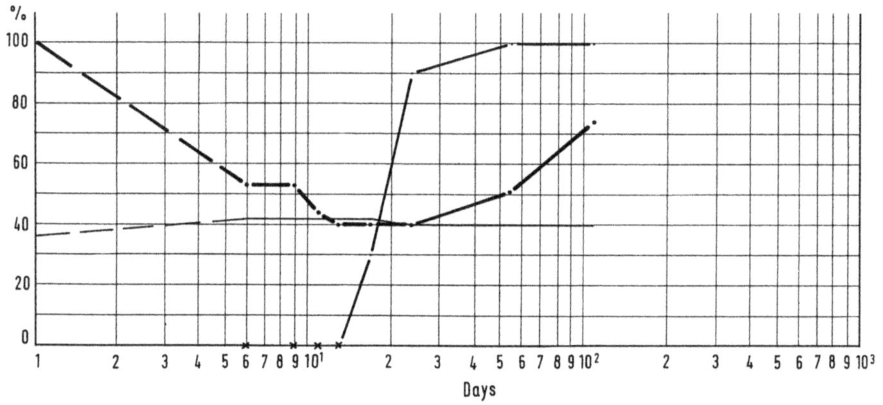

Case 59

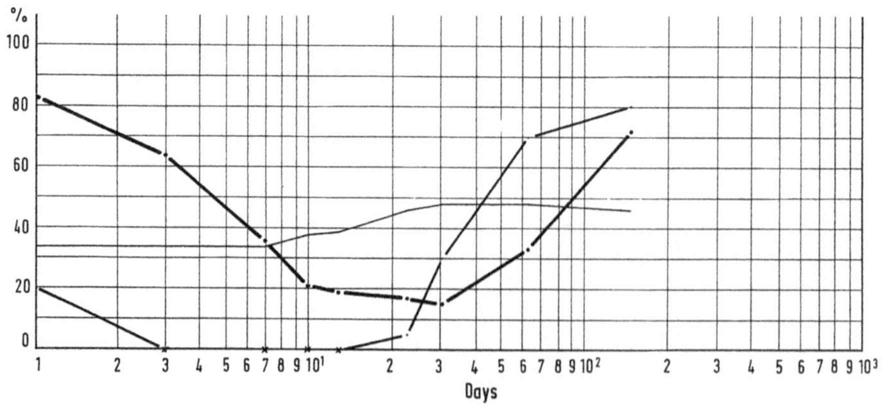

Case 67

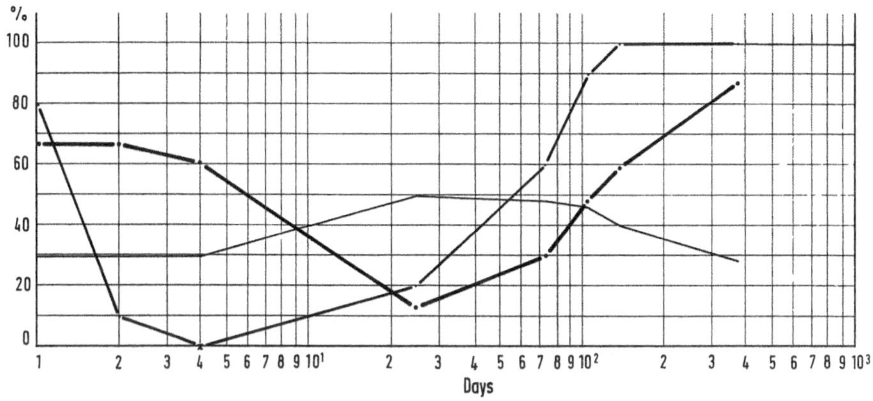

Case 68

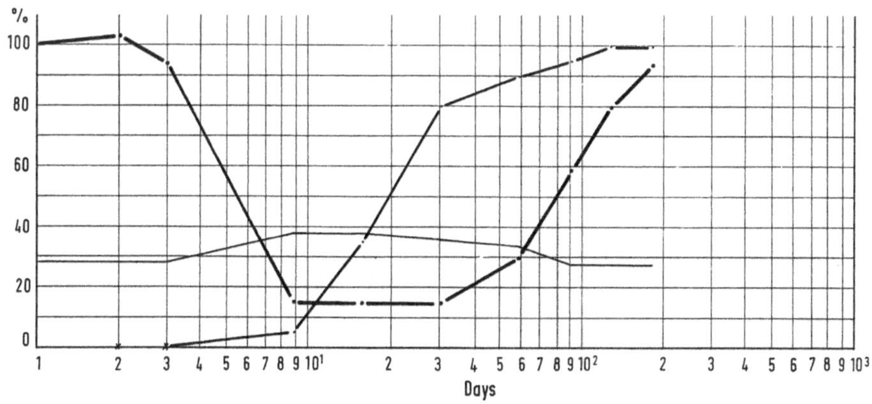

Case 69

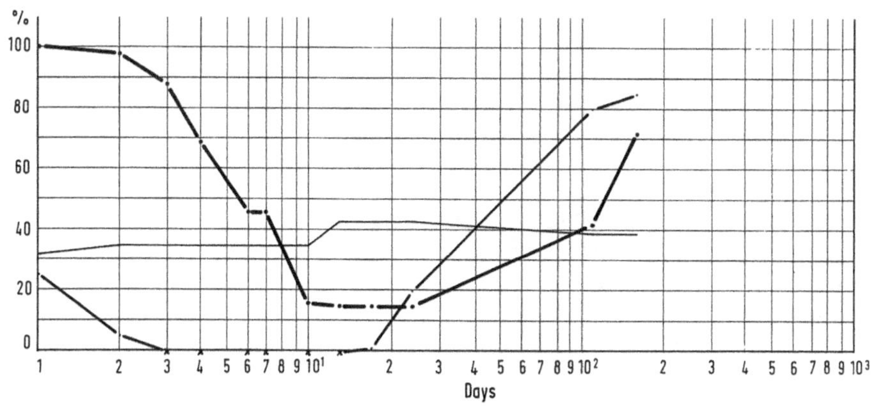

Case 70

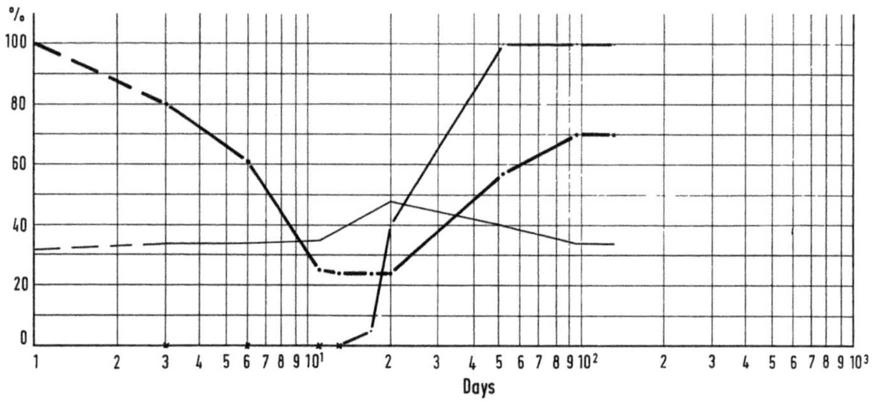

Case 71

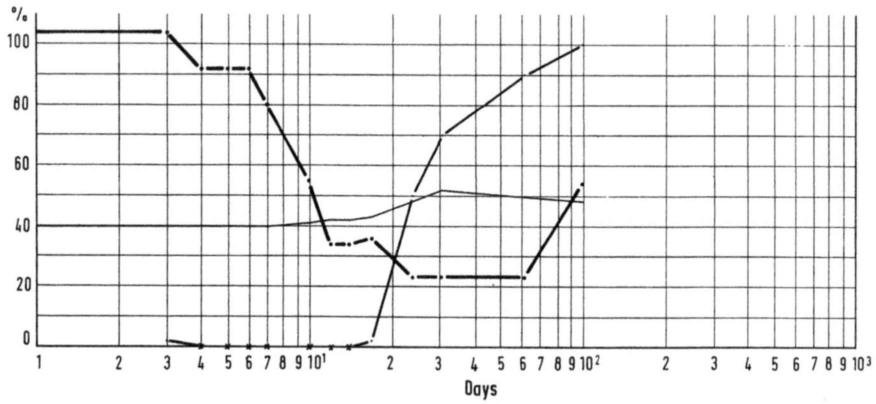

Case 72

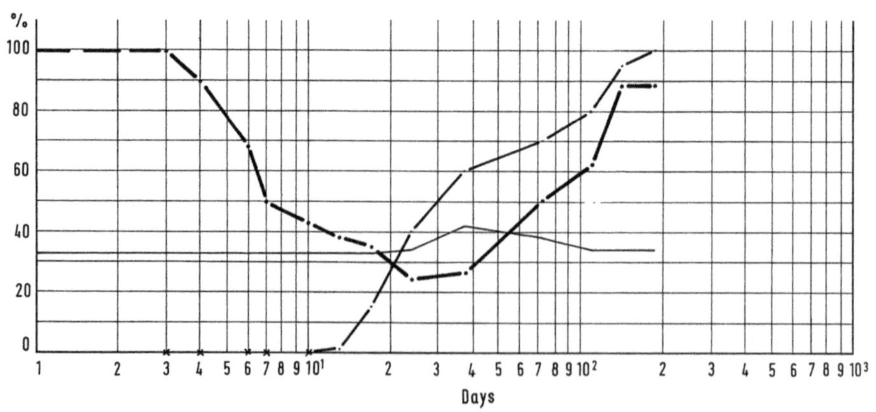

Case 73

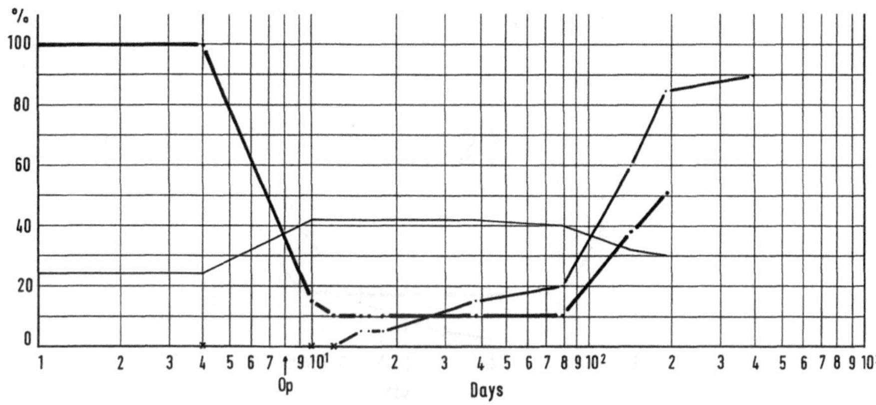

Case 80

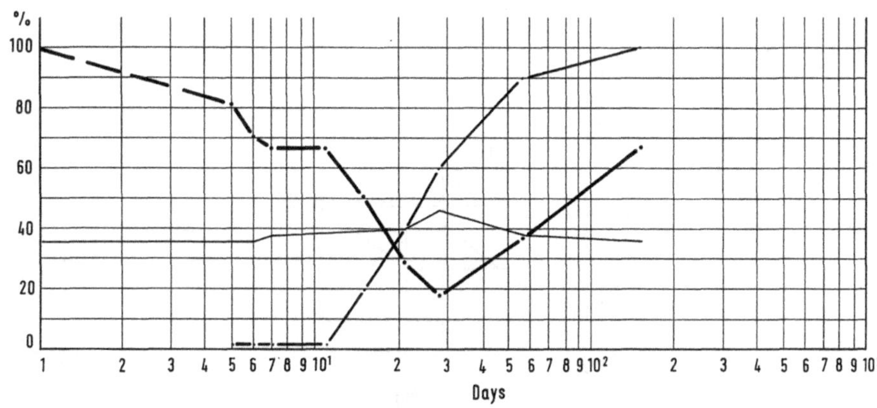

Case 84

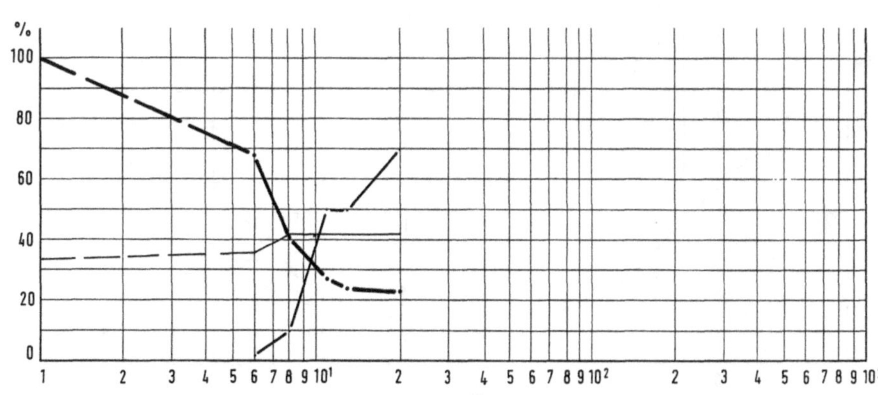

Case 88

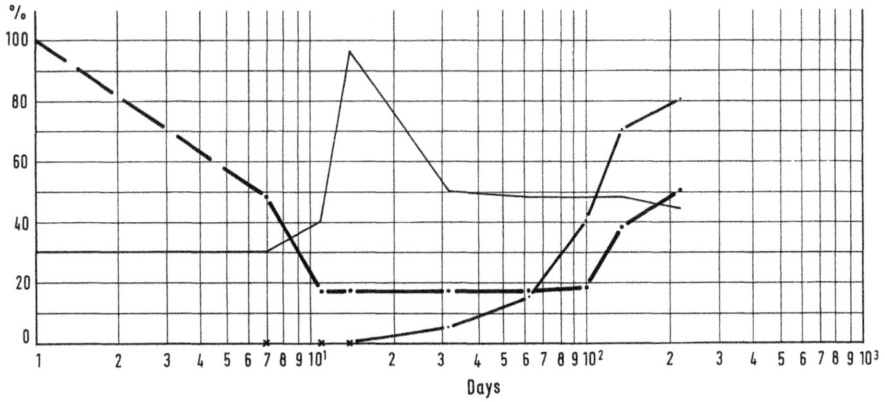

Case 92

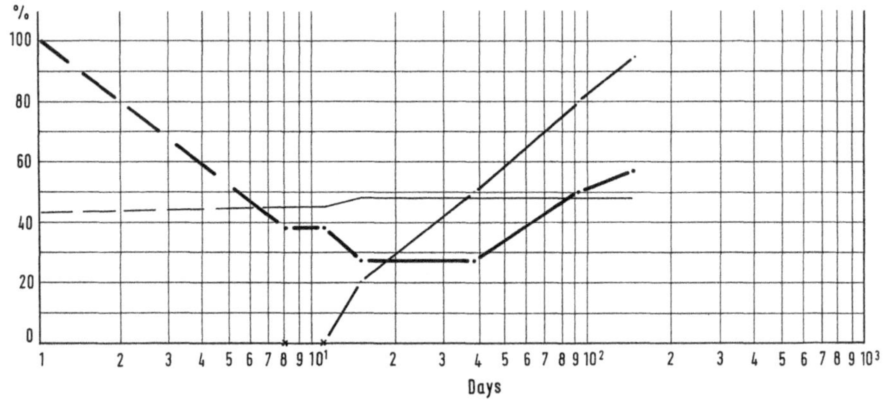

Case 94

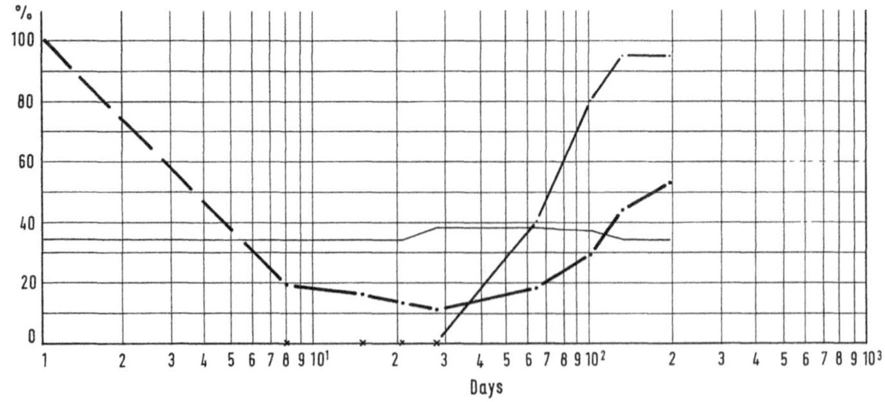

Case 95

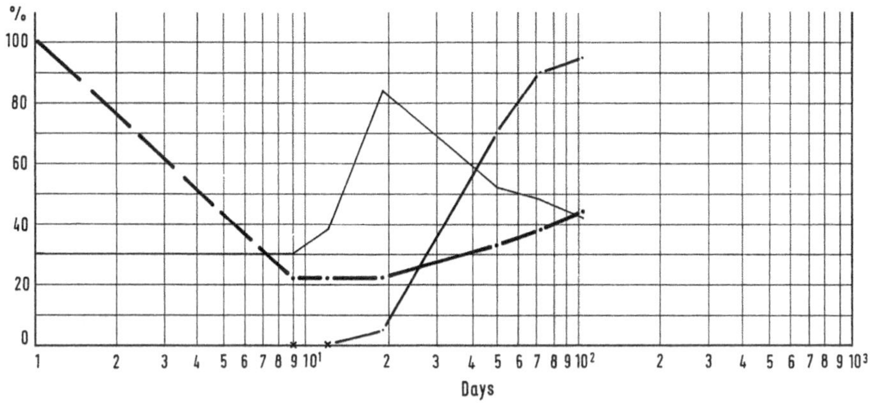

Case 97

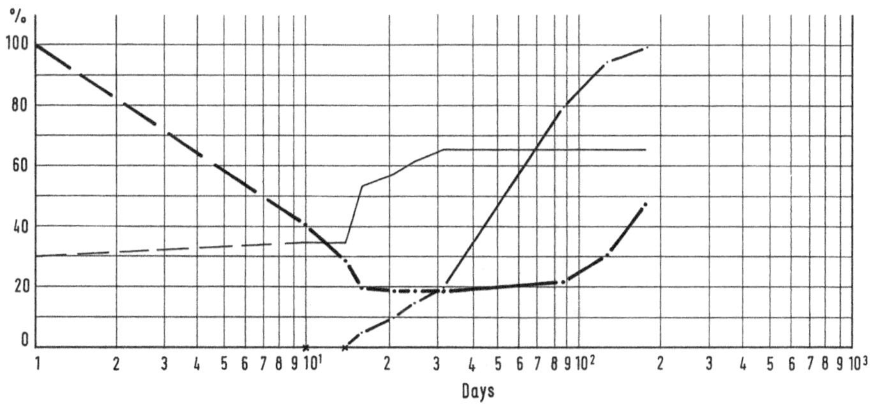

Case 98

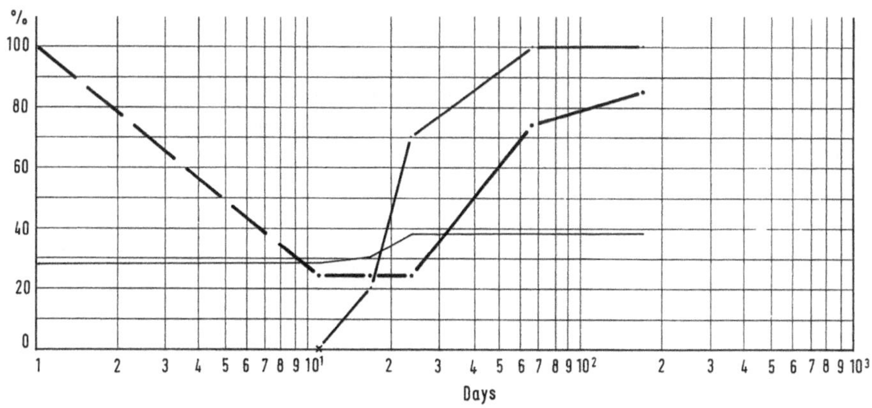

Case 99

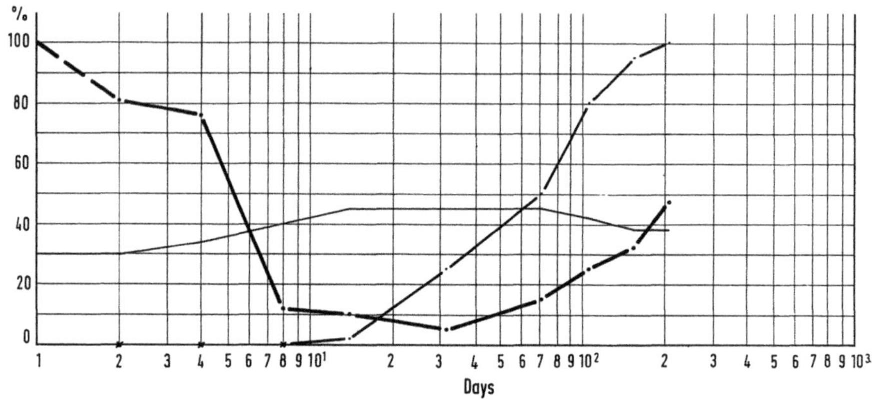

Case 101

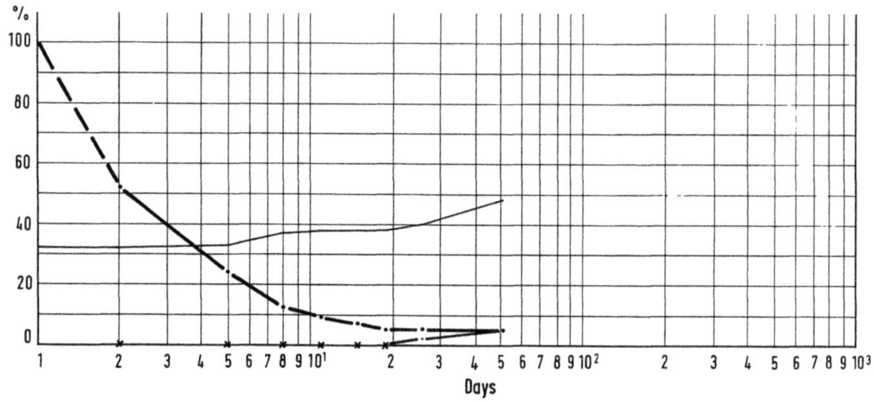

Case 102

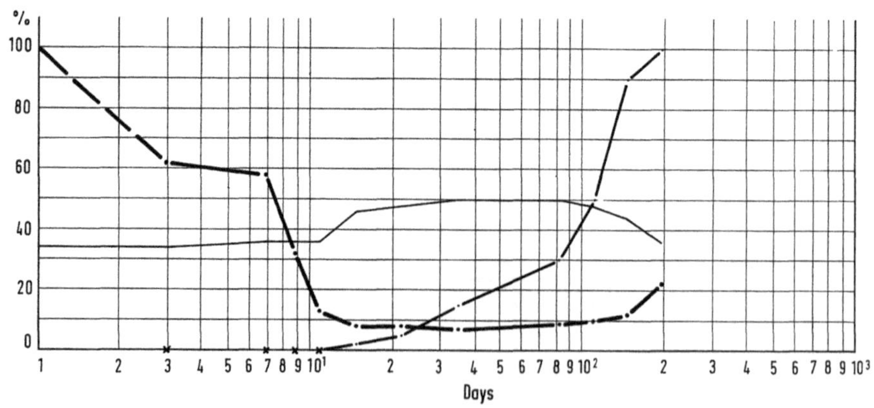

Case 103

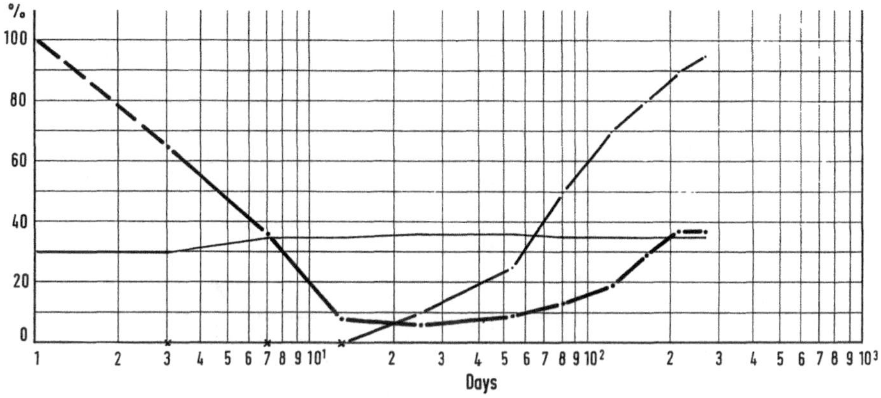

Case 104

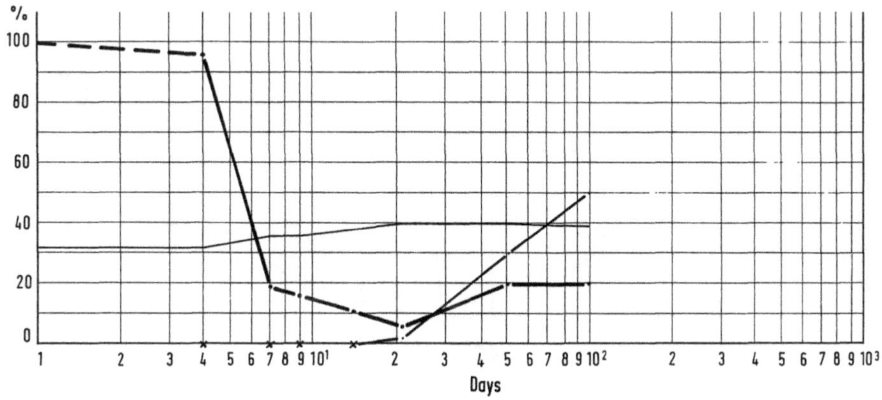

Case 105

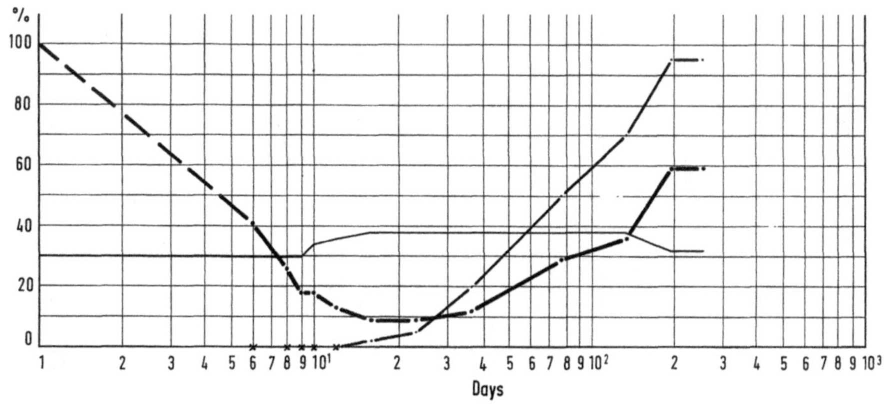

Case 106

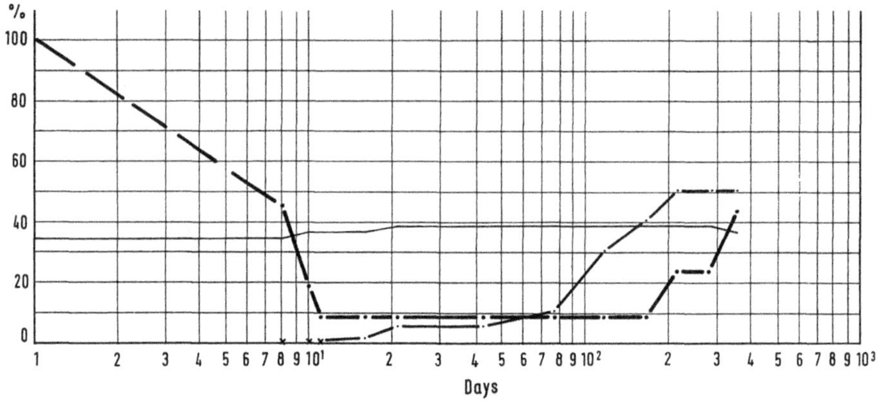

Case 108

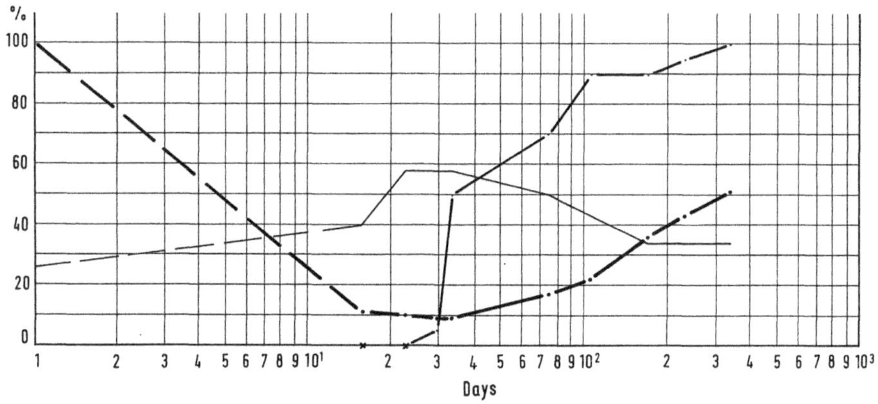

Case 110

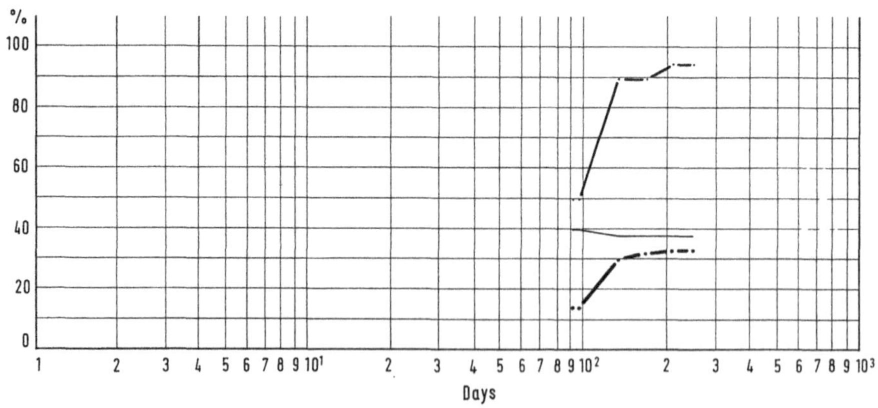

Case 112

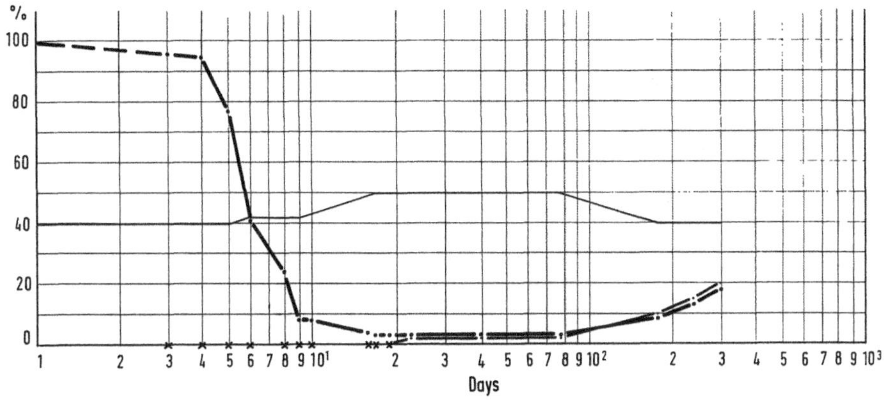

Case 113

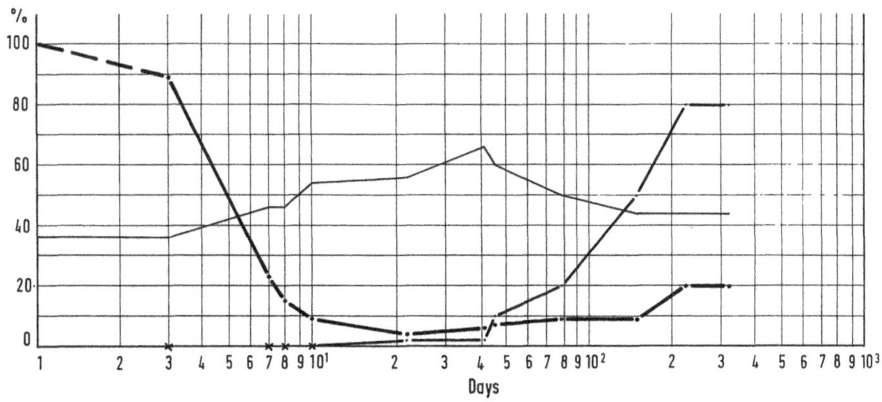

Case 114

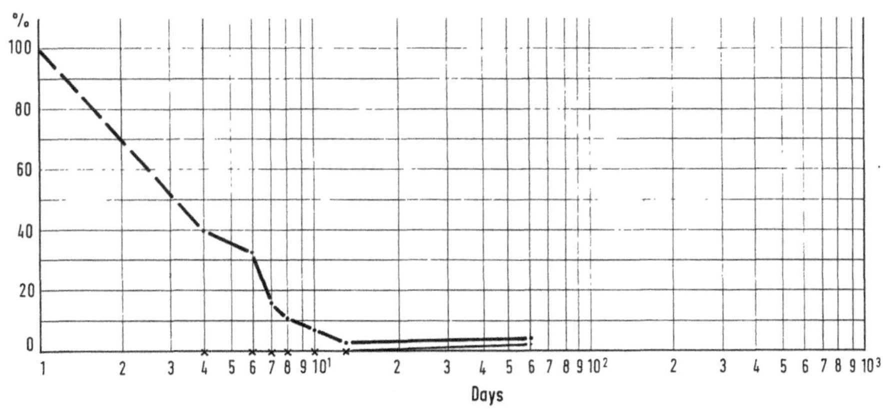

Case 115

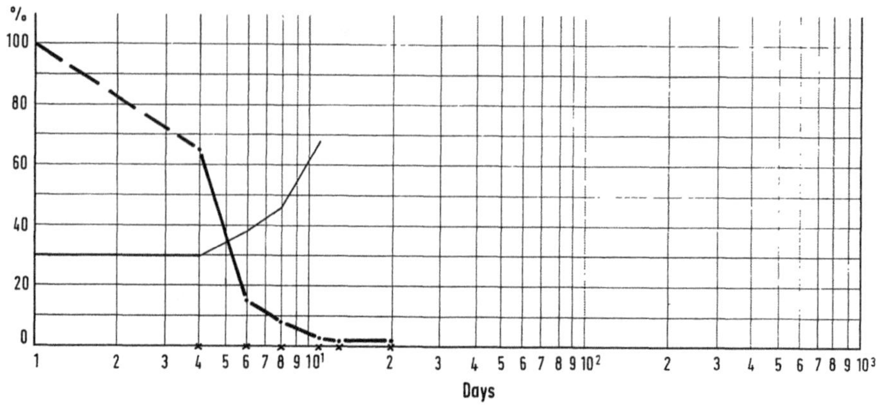

Case 116

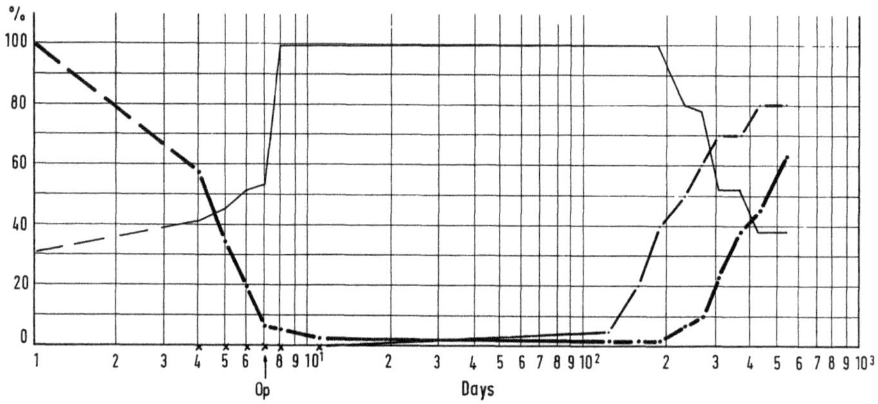

Case 117

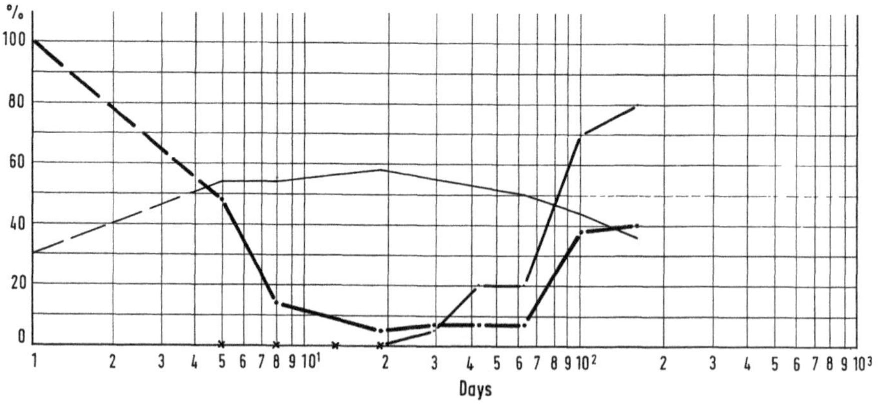

Case 118

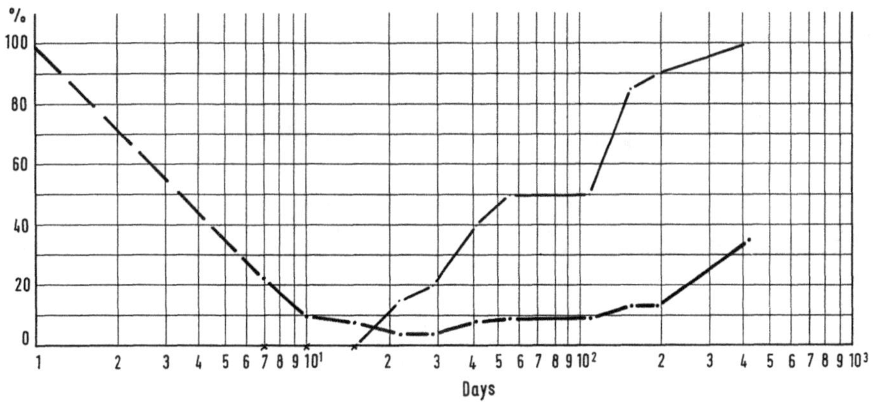

Case 121

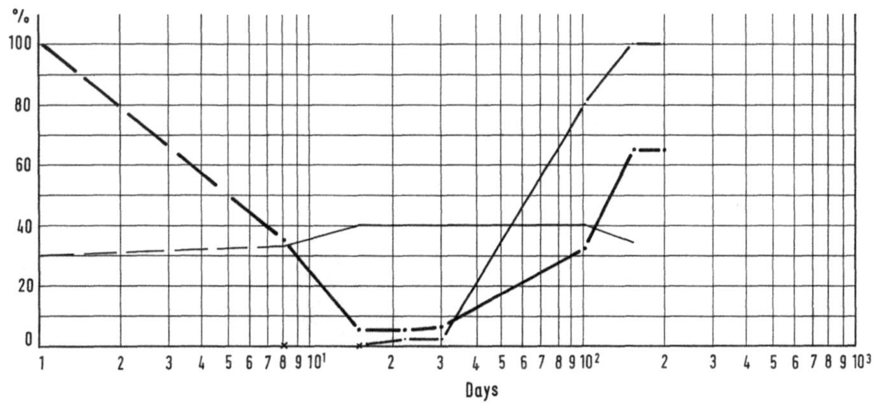

Case 122

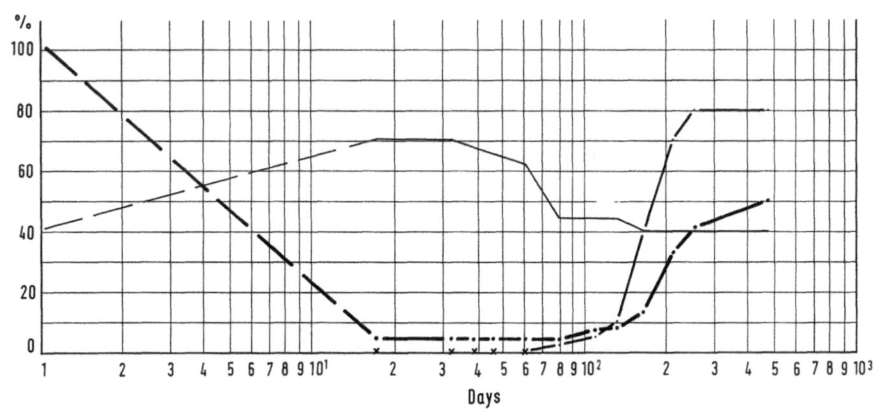

Case 124

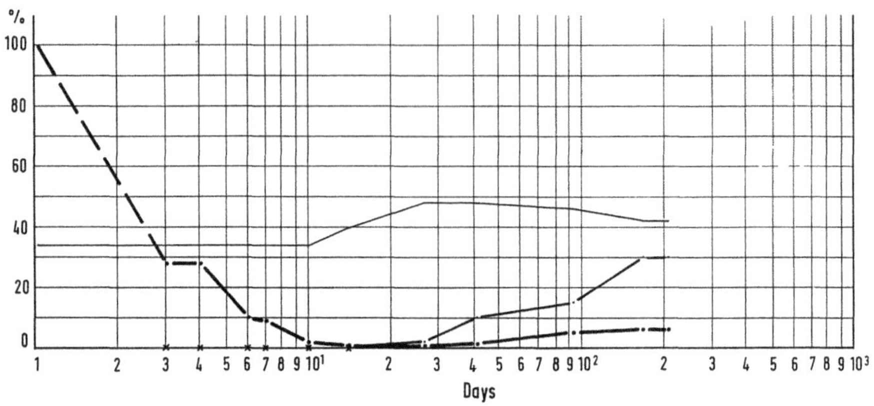

Case 128

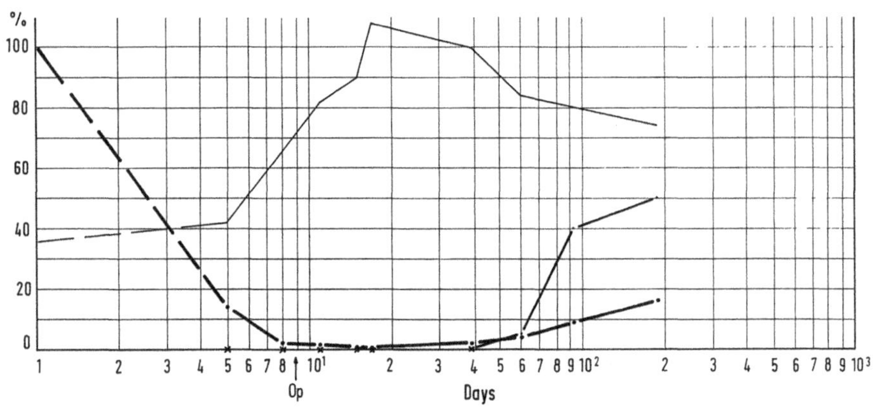

Case 129

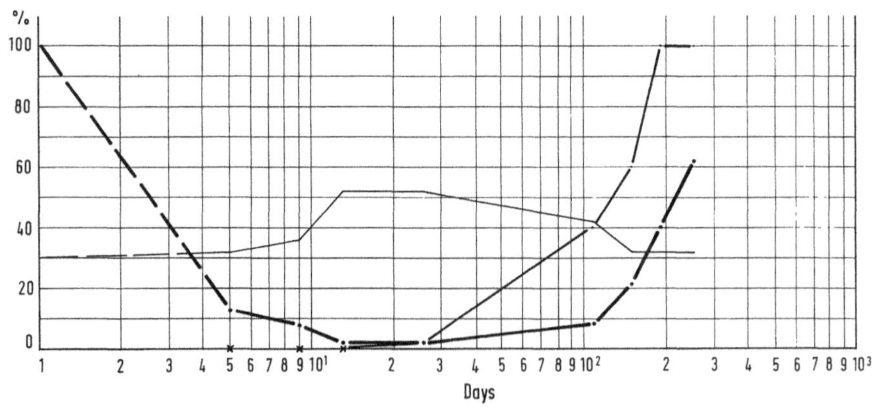

Case 130

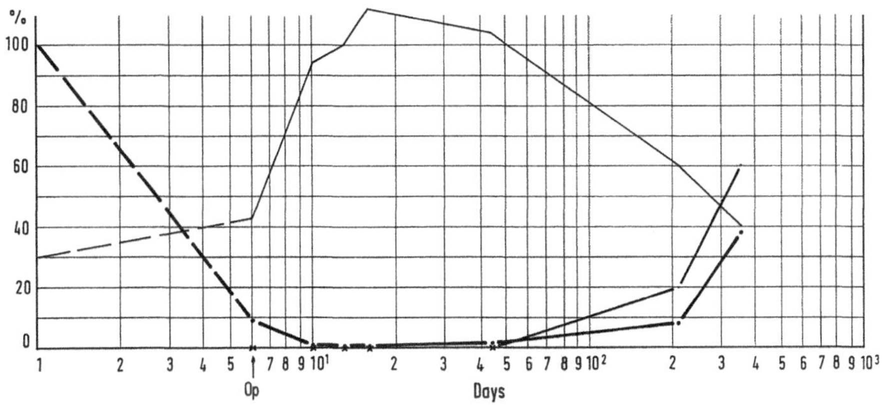

Case 131

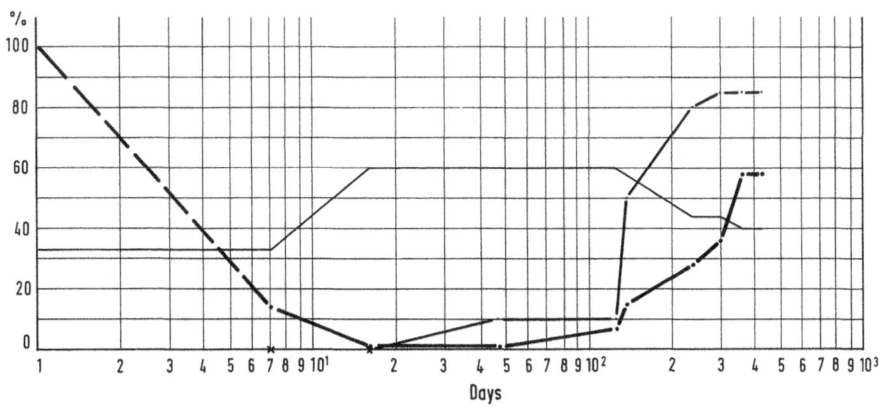

Case 132

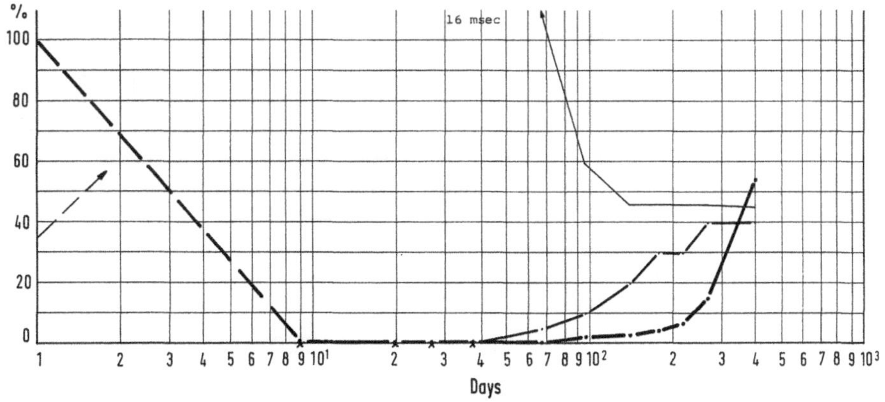

Case 133

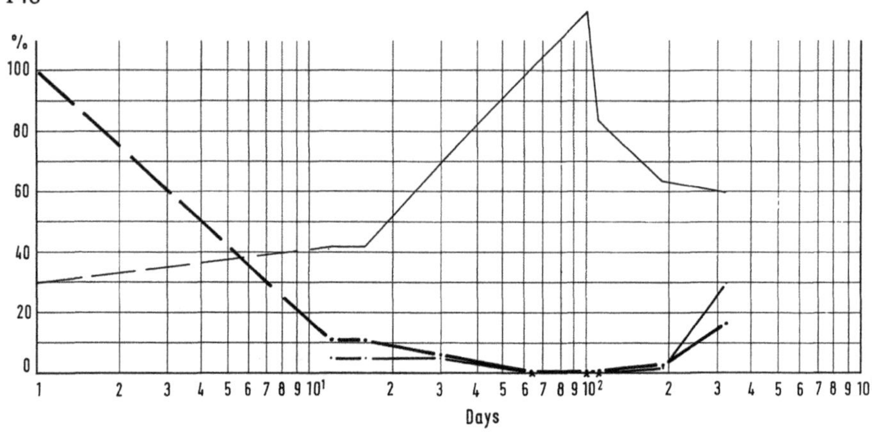

Case 134

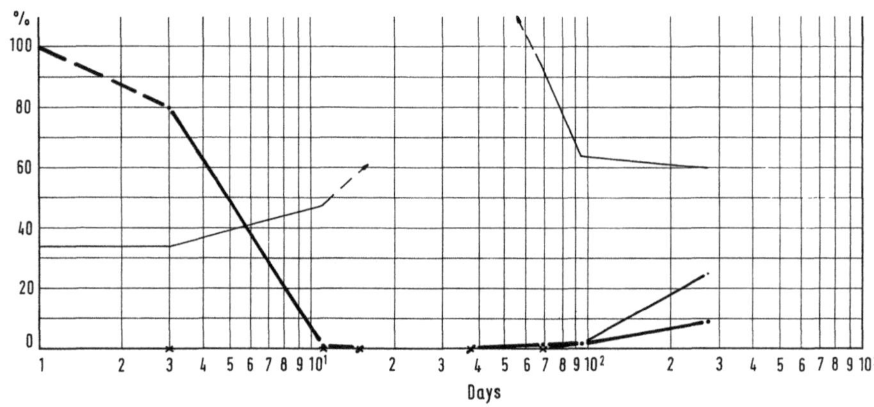

Case 137

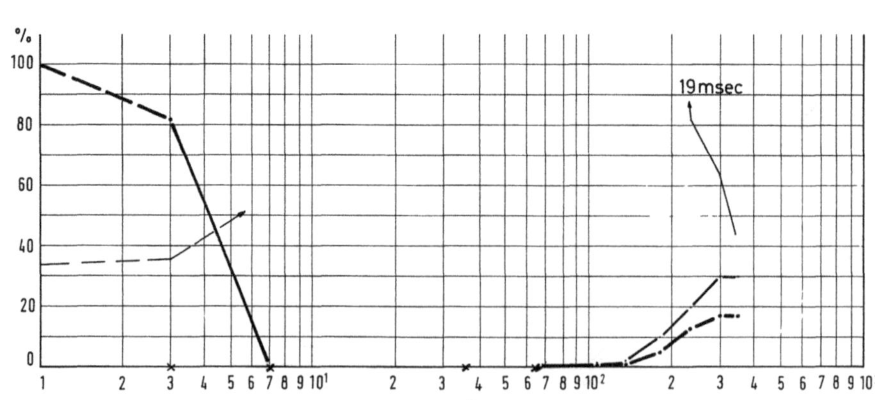

Case 138

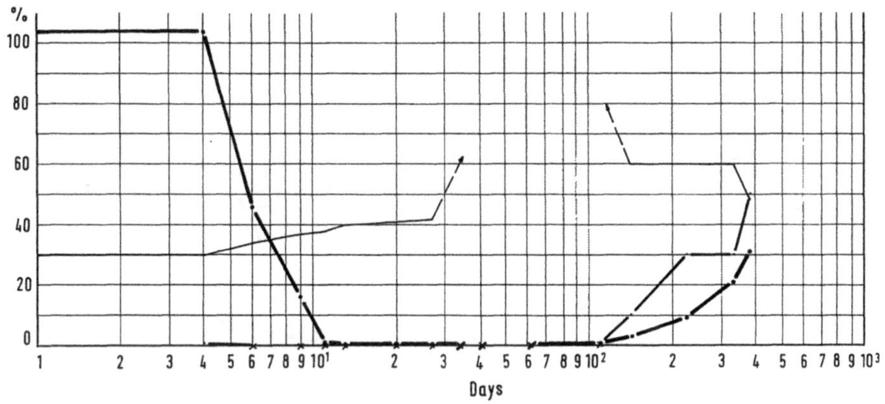

Case 139

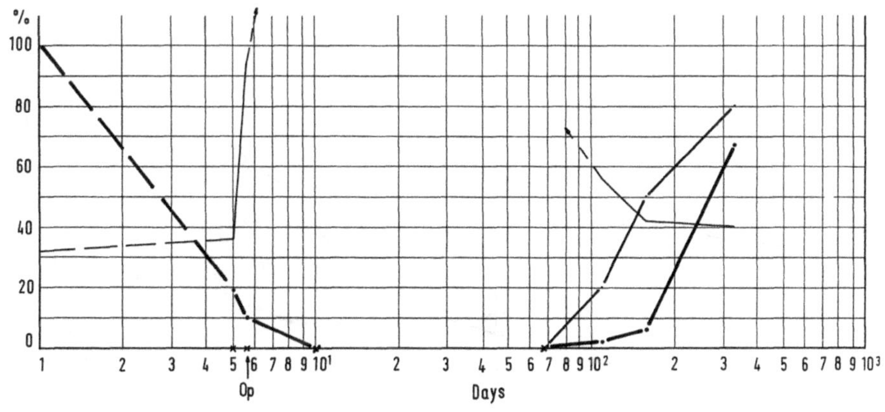

Case 140

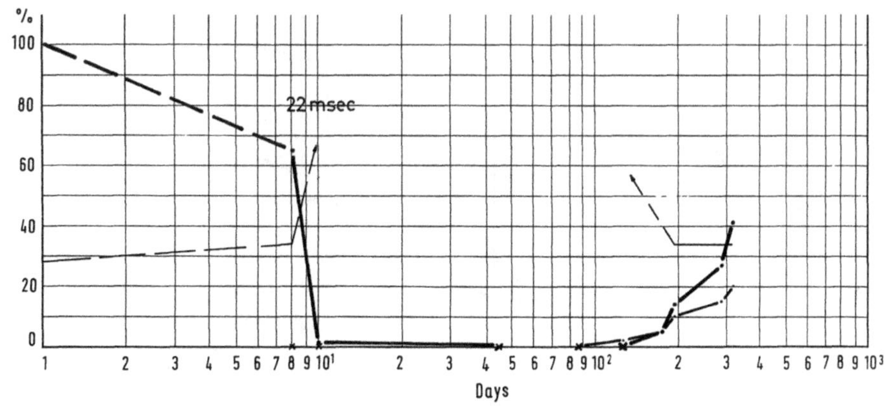

Case 141

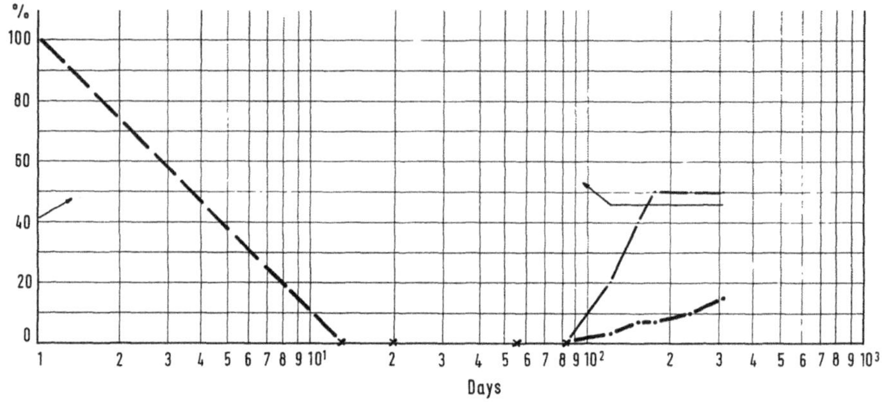

Case 142

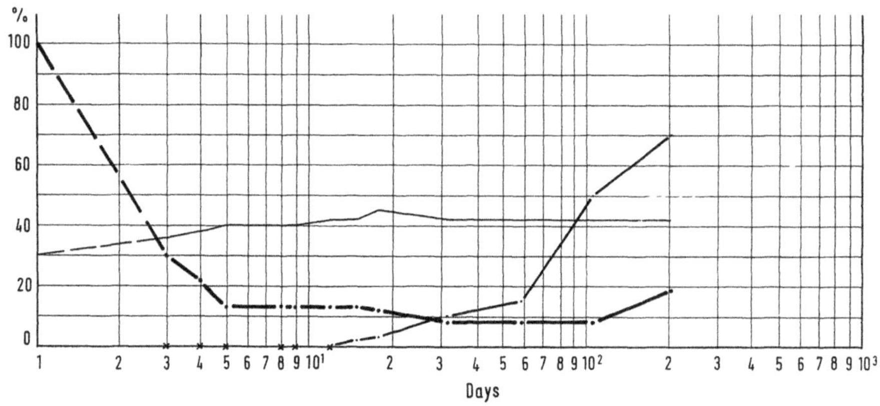

Case Z1

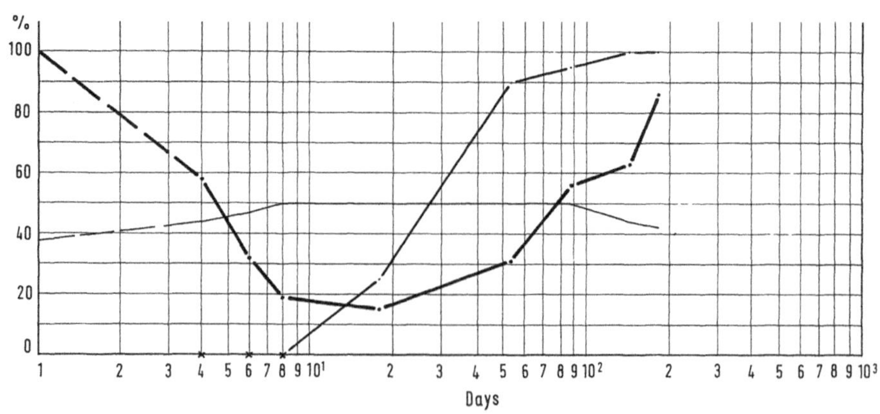

Case Z2

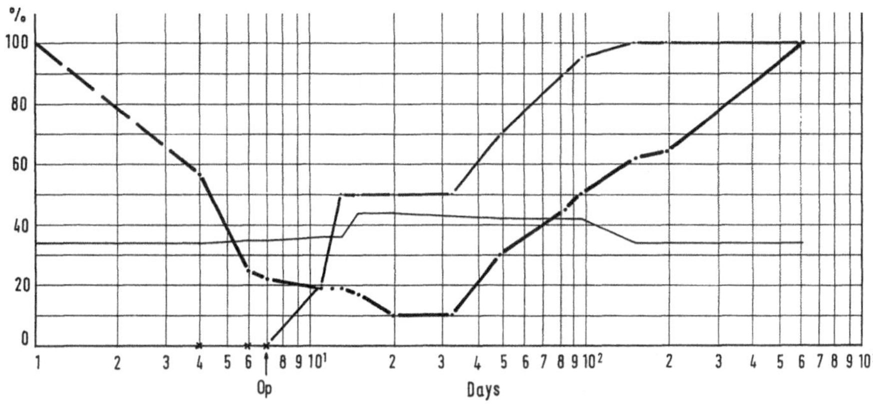

Case Z3

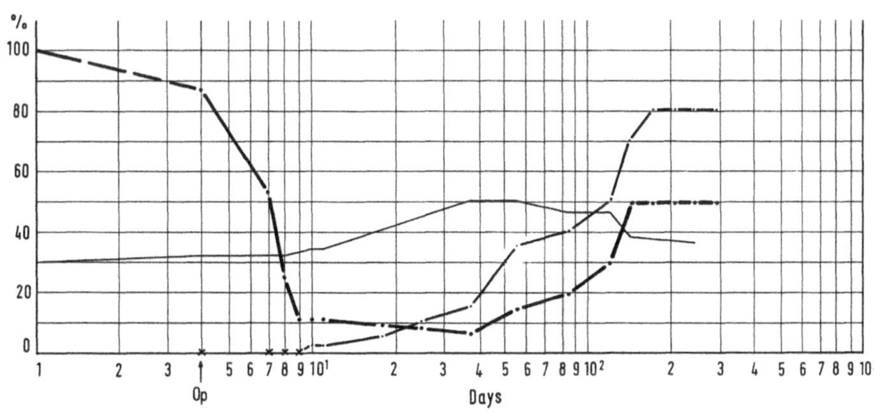

Case Z4

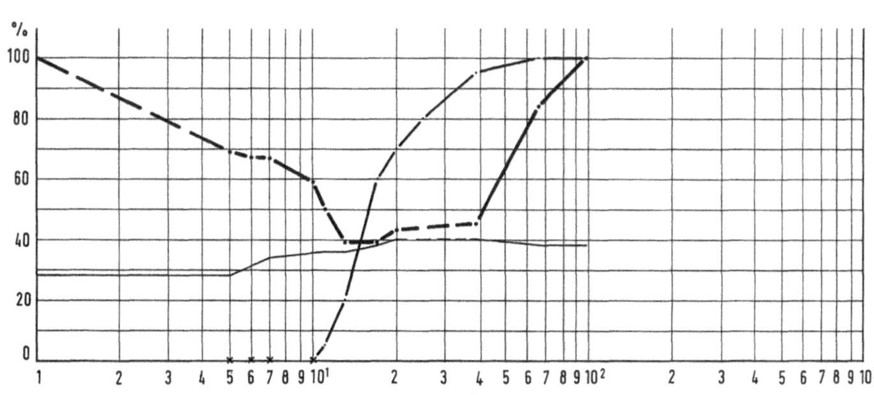

Case Z5

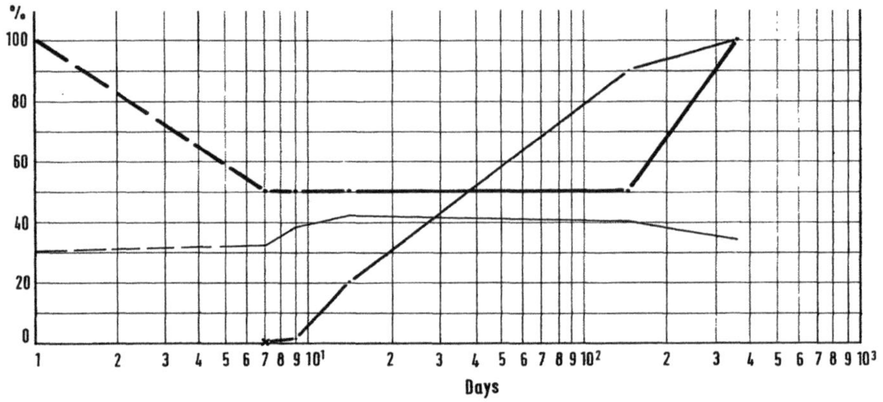

Case Z6

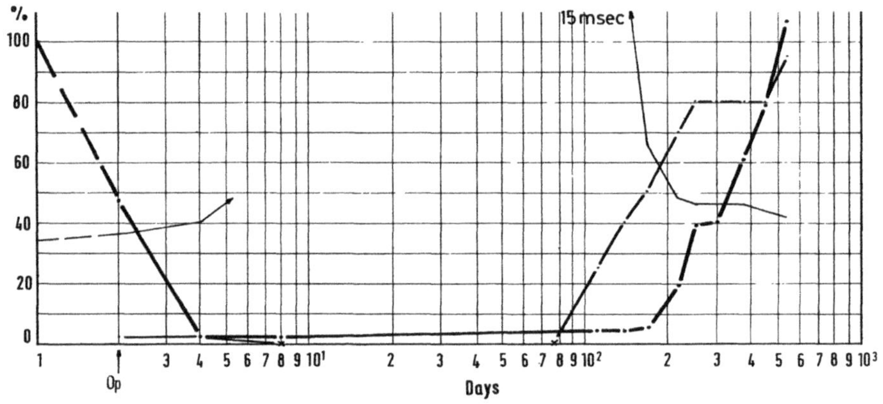

Case Z8

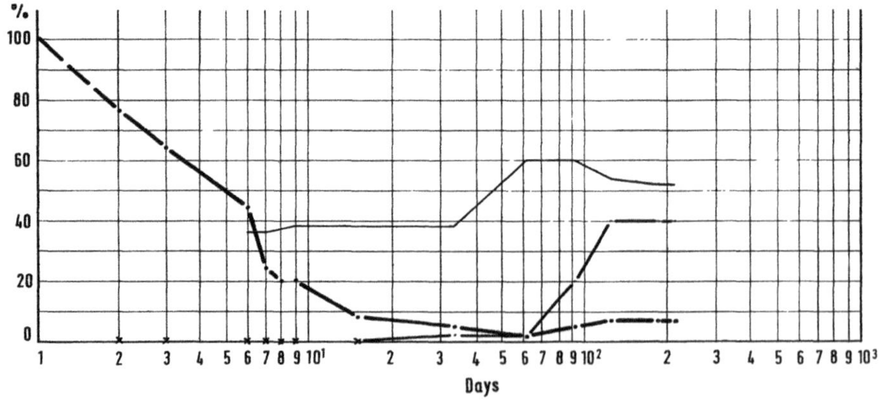

Case Z9

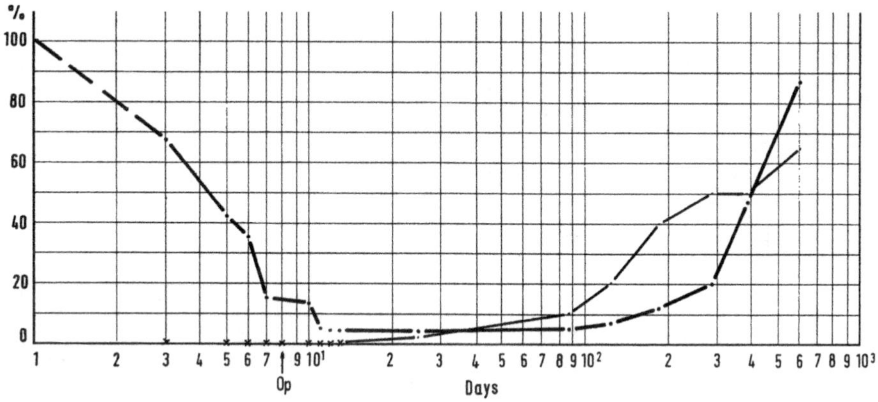

Case Z10

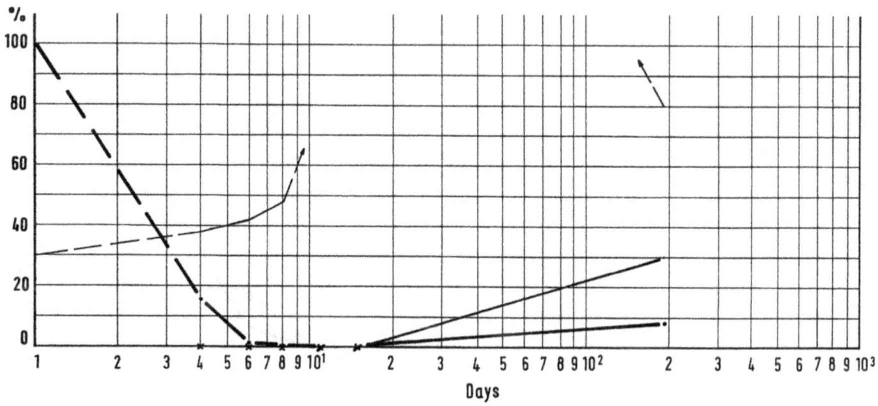

Case Z11

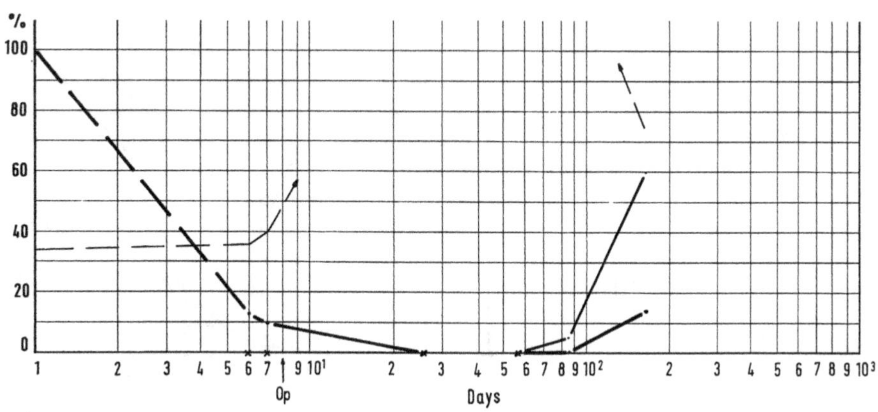

Case Z12

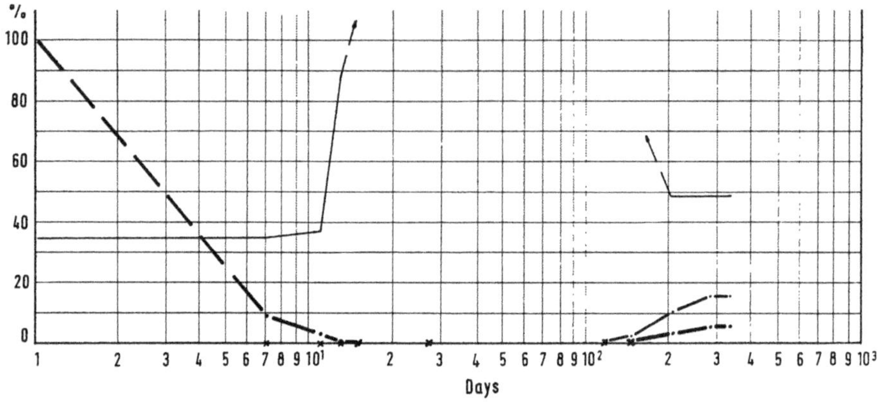

Case Z13

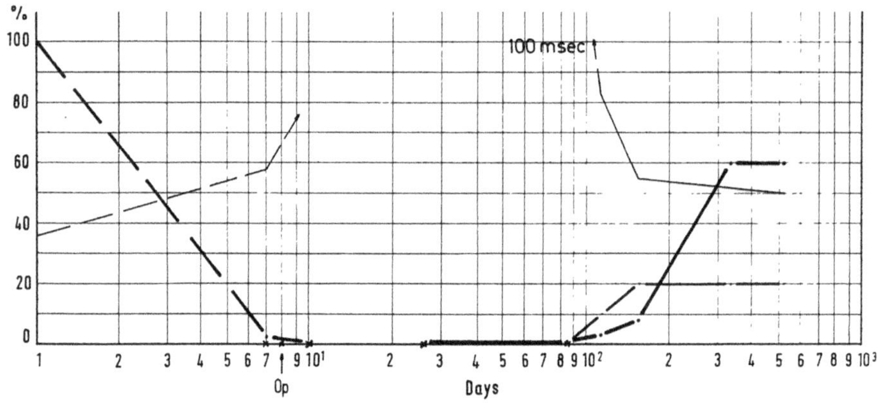

Case Z14

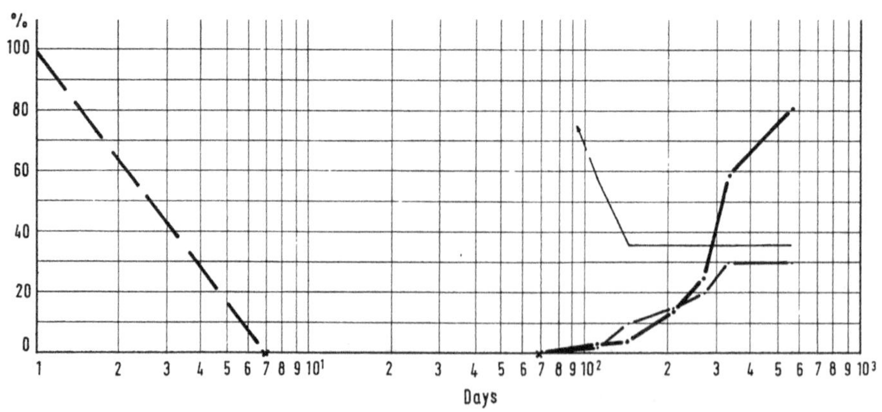

Case Z15

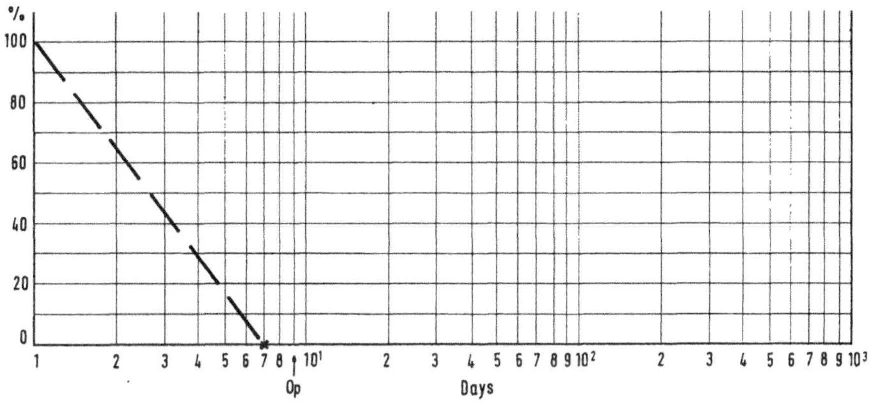

Case Z16

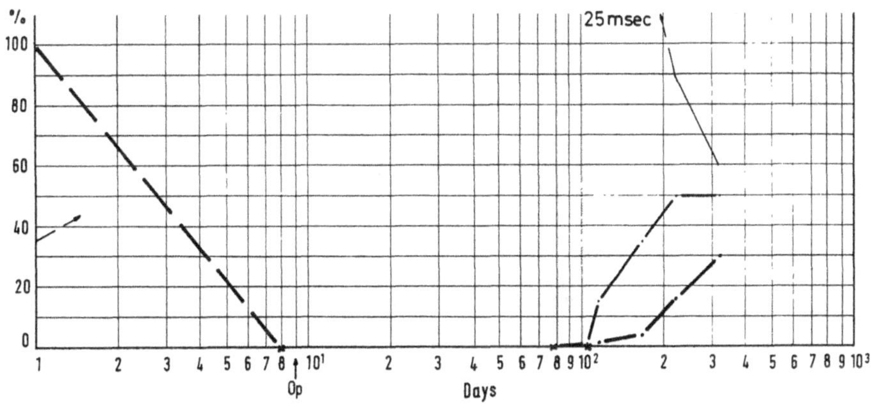

Case Z17

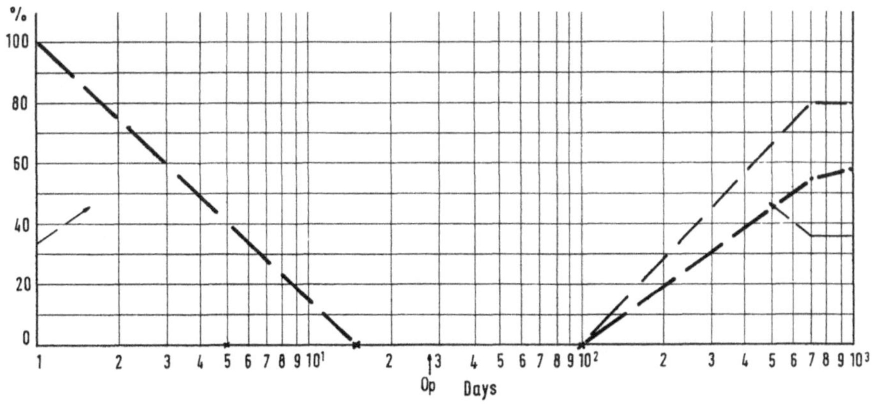

Case Z19

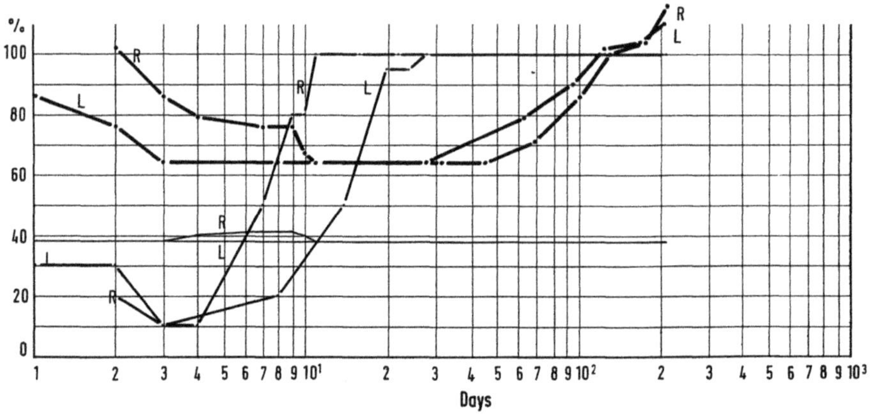

Case B1 (105)

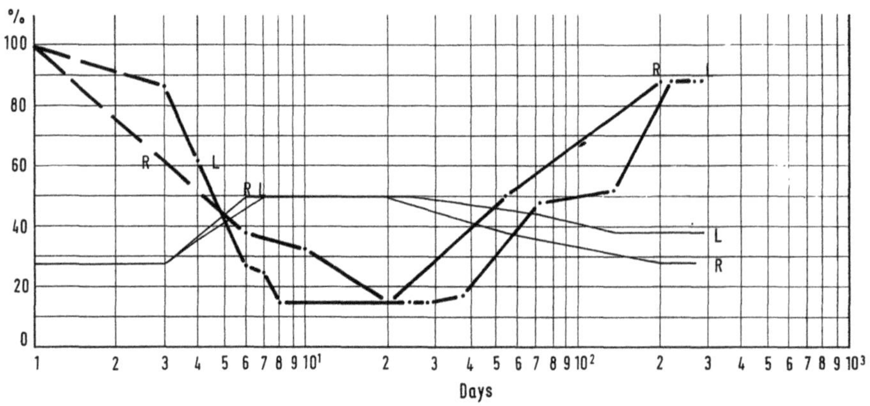

Case B2 (106)

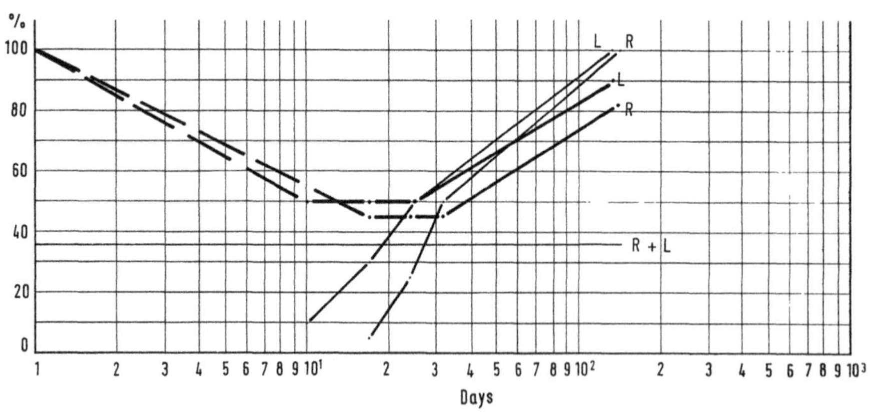

Case B3 (107)

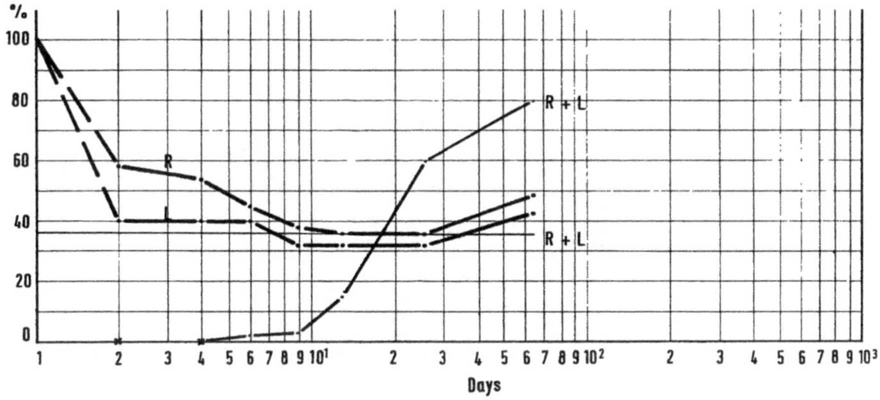

Case B4

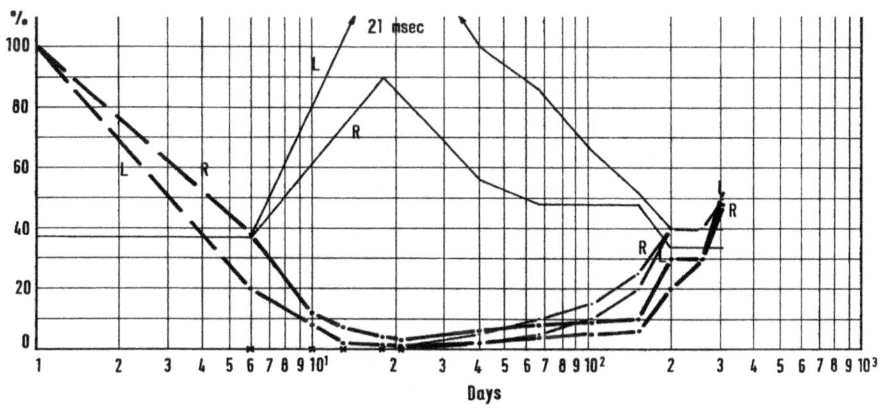

Case B5

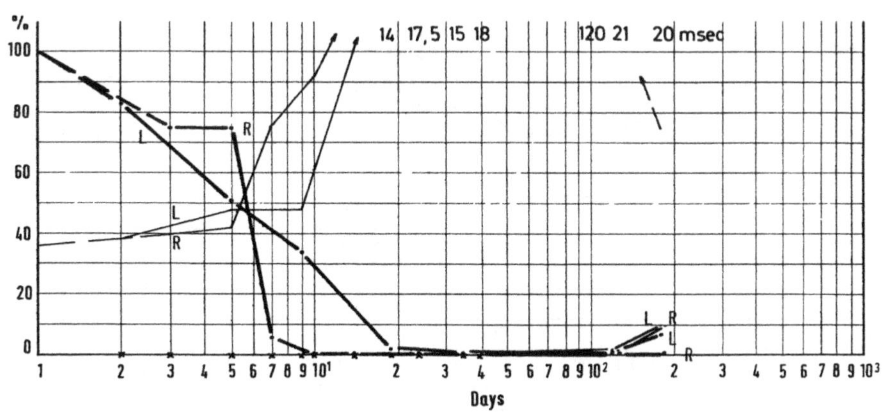

Case B6

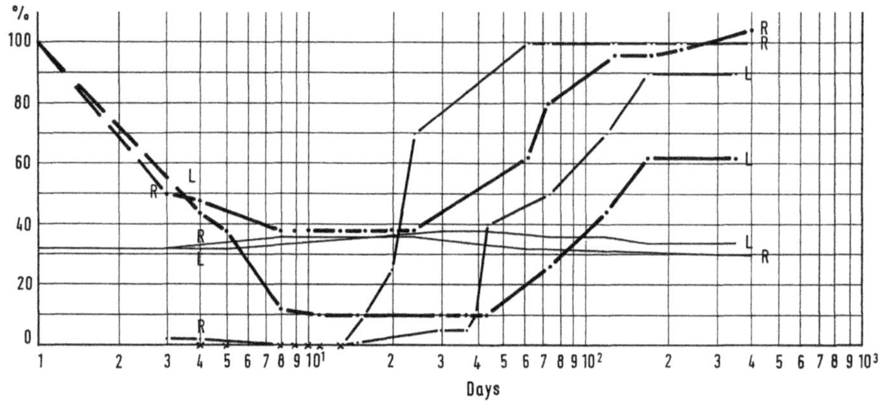

Case B7

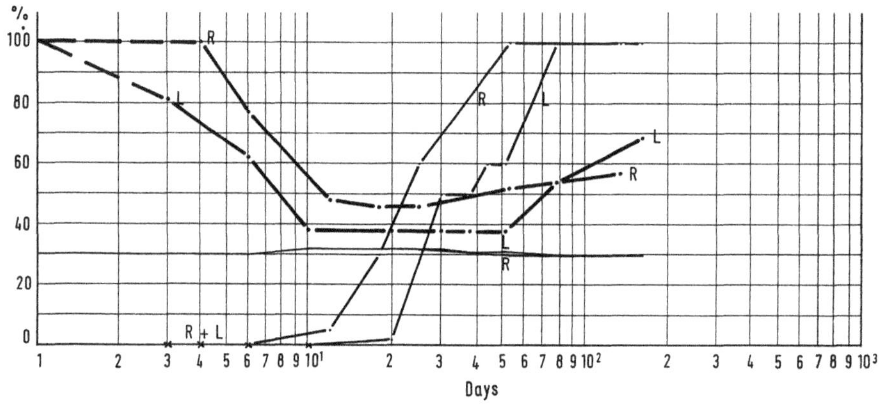

Case B8

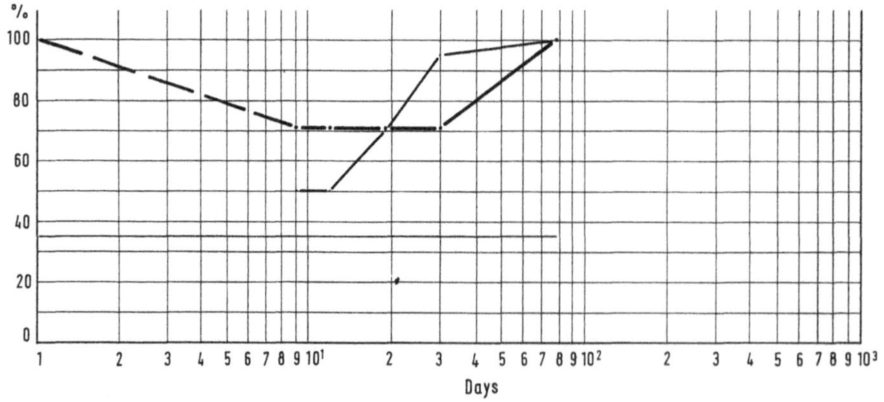

Case V1

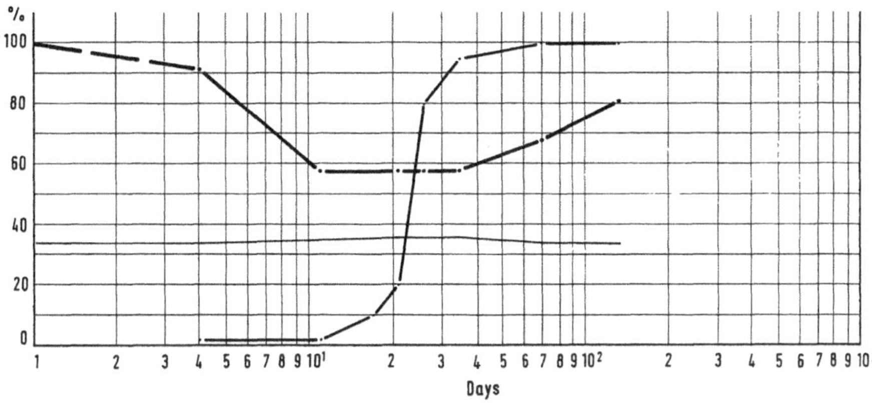

Case V2

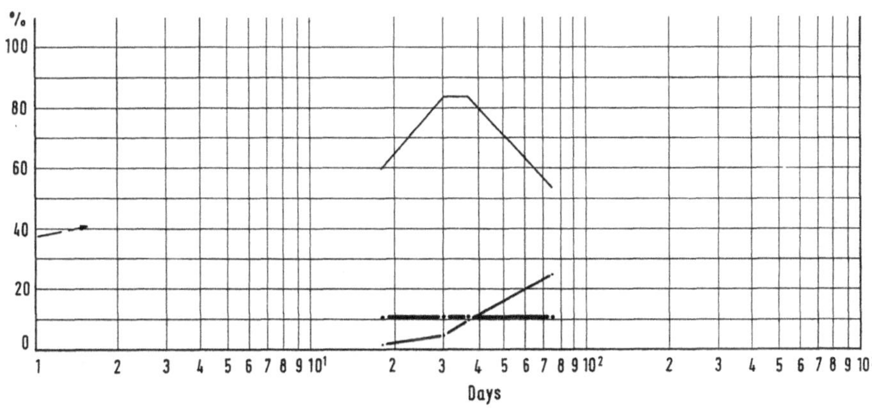

Case V3

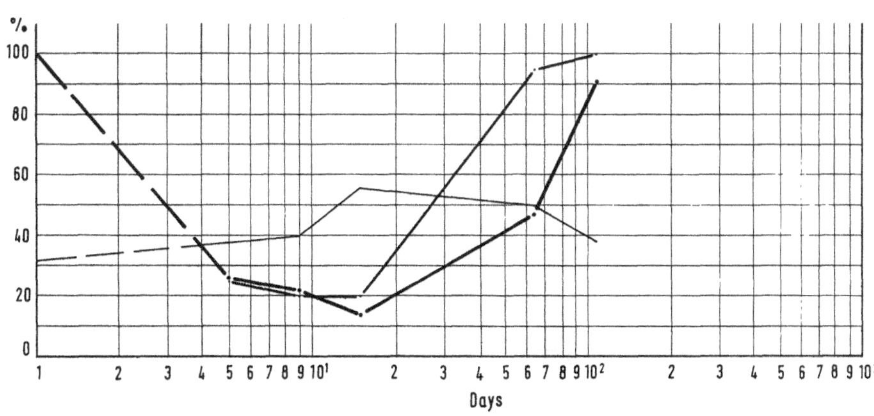

Case V4

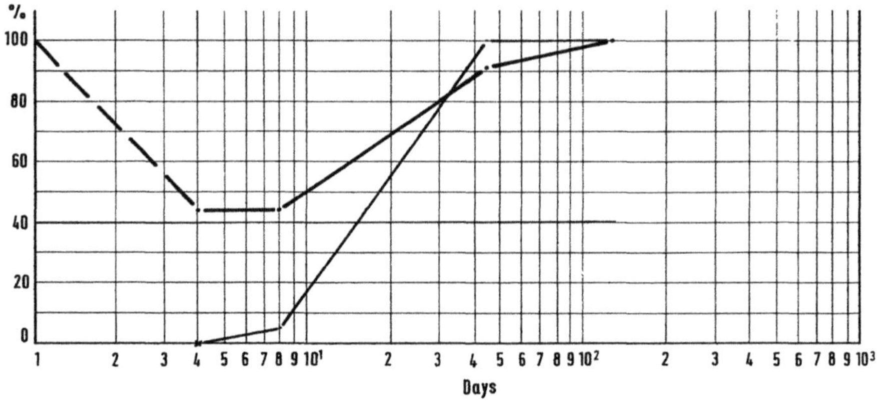

Case V5

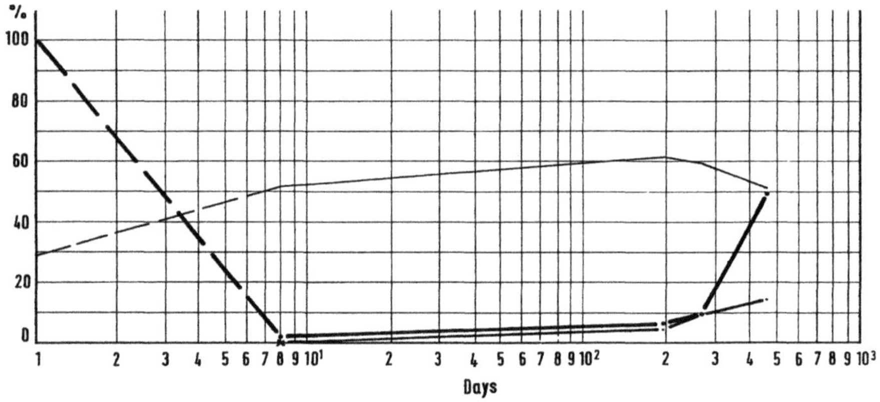

Case V6

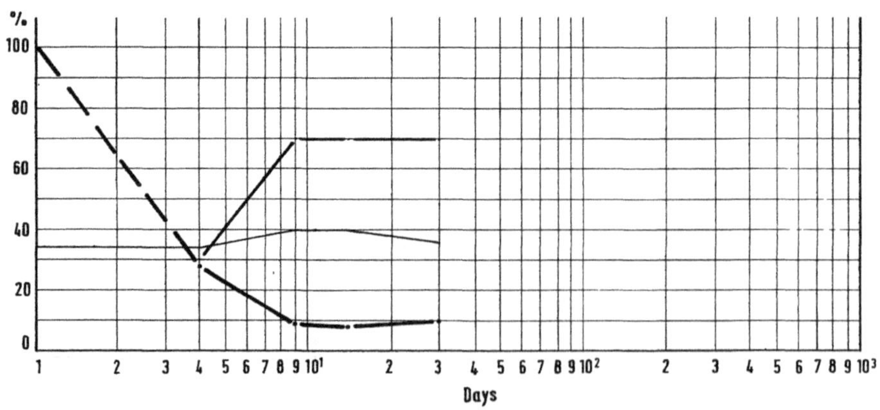

Case V7

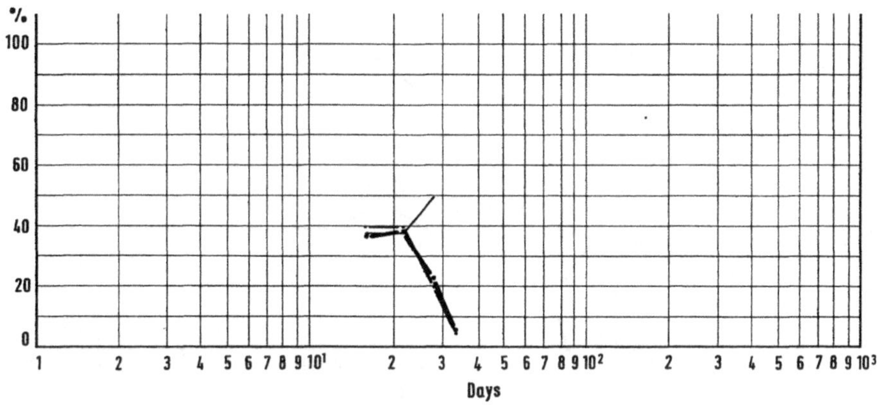

Case V8

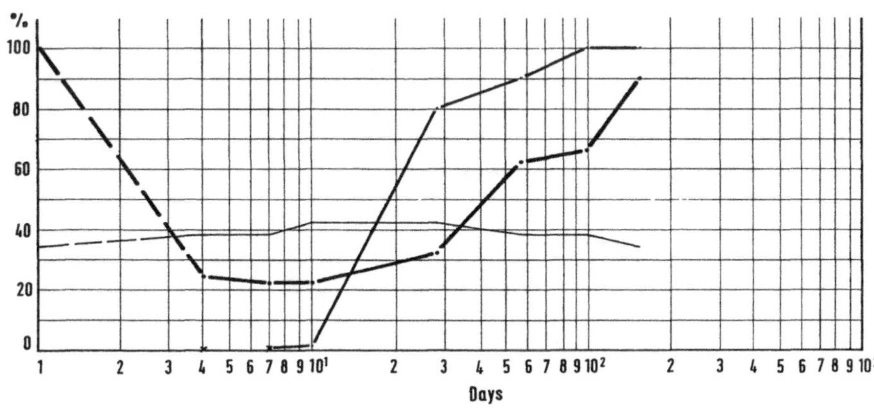

Case T1

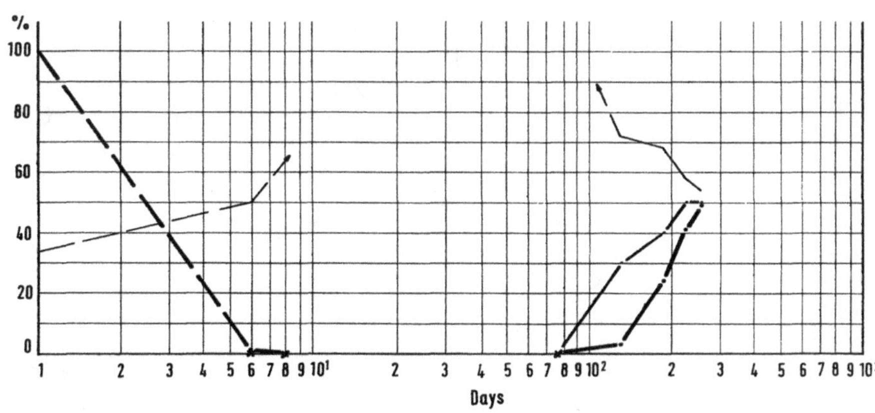

Case T2

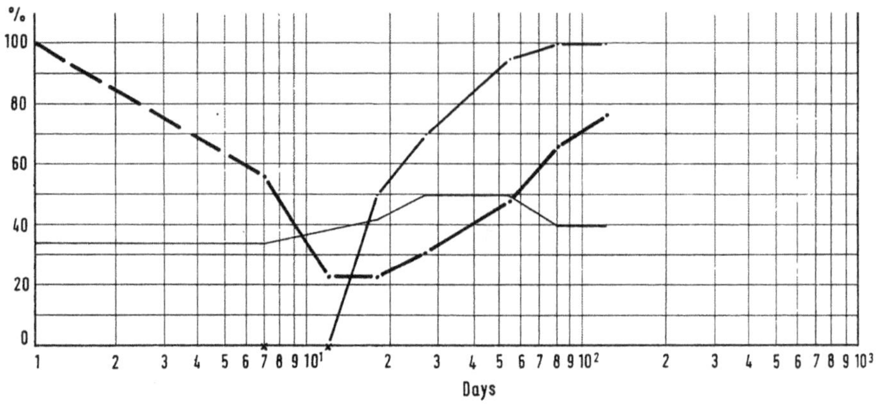

Case T3

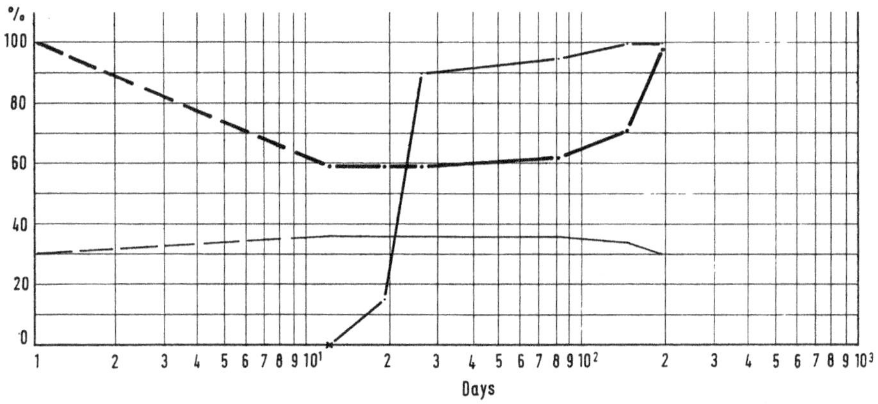

Case T4

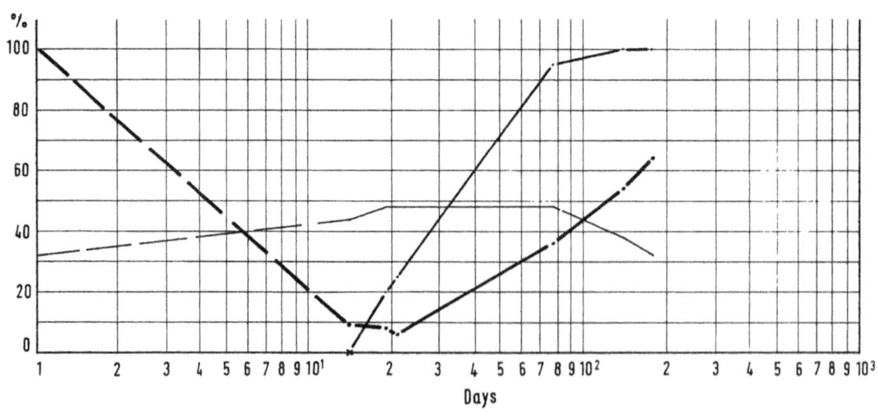

Case T5

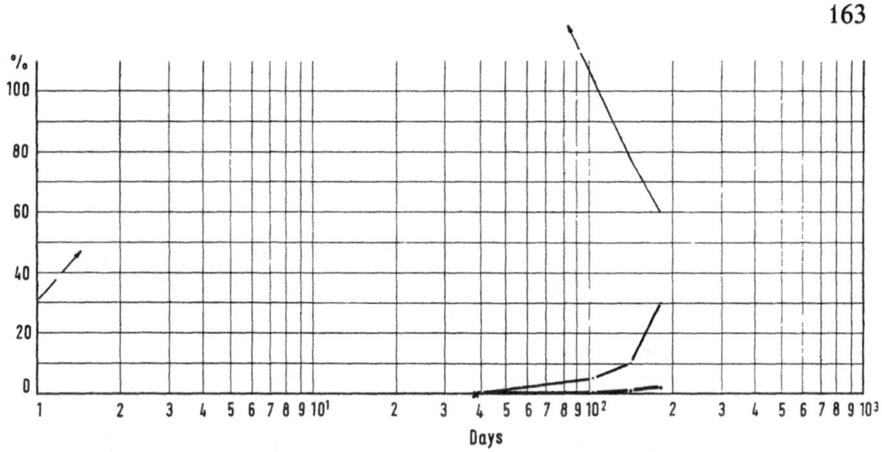

Case T6

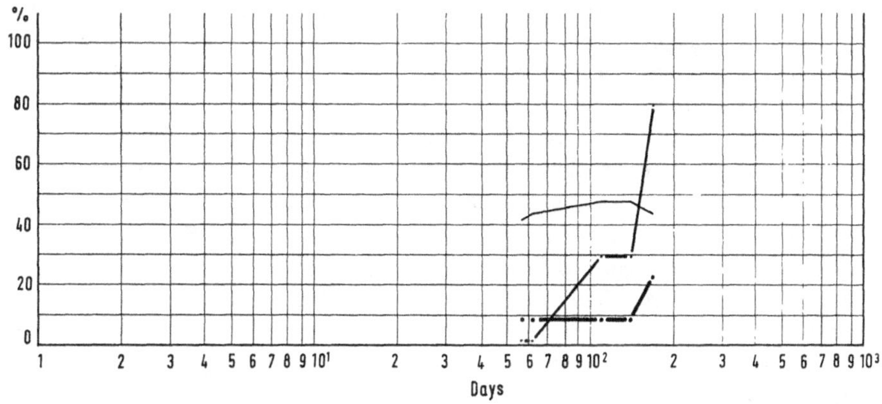

Case T7

Author's Postscript

Unforeseen events have delayed publication of this monograph. The experience gathered in the meantime has provided ample opportunity to validate the statements made here. On the other hand, most of the open questions still have found no answer. Experimental models to produce and study facial palsy have until now been designed to reproduce vasoconstriction and primary ischemia of the nerve within its canal. The essential question, however, is no longer what causes vasoconstriction in the canal but what initiates vasodilation, increase of vascular permeability and hemorrhage of facial nerve vessels at the entrance. A tempting explanation is to think in terms of an immune reaction causing vasodilation by inflammatory mediators (histamine, etc). But then a cellular inflammatory reaction should be expected.

Unfortunately, the available histopathologic evidence is not sufficient to answer the question definitely one way or the other. In the case cited by Proctor et al. (1976) in which autopsy was performed on the 11th day of palsy there were some signs of inflammation, specific or not. In Fowler's case, autopsied after 14 days of palsy, no signs of inflammation could be observed (cf. pp. 27–29). Experimental work on animals has proved that in an originally cellular inflammatory immune reaction all cellular elements may disappear within 8–10 days. Therefore neither the case of Proctor nor that of Fowler can settle this question and we shall have to wait until the opportunity comes for histological examination of the *whole* nerve during the first week of palsy.

But it is even more urgent to find an acceptable solution to the therapeutic problem. The skill and precision required in transtemporal decompression of the facial nerve may be technically fascinating, but the method is no substitute for an effective non-operative treatment. One hundred cases, on prednisolone from the *very* beginning and controlled by electroneurographic technique, could perhaps solve the problem. The doses would need to be high enough, at least 60 mg prednisolone during the first 4 days, then 40 mg until day 7 and 30 mg until day 10.

V. Chan-Palay

Cerebellar Dentate Nucleus

Organization, Cytology, and Transmitters
293 figures, including 79 plates, some in color. Approx. 600 pages. 1977. ISBN 3-540-07958-0

G. Salamon, Y. P. Huang

Radiologic Anatomy of the Brain

In cooperation with P. Michotoy, N. Moscow, C. Raybaud, P. Farnarier, G. Scialfa, W. O. Bank, K. Hall, B. S. Wolf, T. Okudera, K. Oana, S. Panichavatena, J. Ito, R. Kawai, S. Antin, J. Pinner, N. Christoff
282 figures in 463 separate illustrations. XII, 404 pages. 1976. Distribution rights for Japan: Nankodo Co. Ltd. Tokyo. ISBN 3-540-07528-3

B. Schlesinger

The Upper Brainstem in the Human

Its Nuclear Configuration and Vascular Supply.
With a Foreword by H. Ferner.
326 figures, some in color. 10 tables. XVI, 266 pages. 1976. ISBN 3-540-07497-X

H. W. Kölmel

Atlas of Cerebrospinal Fluid Cells

201 figures, 131 in color. VIII, 124 pages. 1976. ISBN 3-540-07607-7

Cerebral Angiomas

Advances in Diagnosis and Therapy
Editors: H. W. Pia, J. R. Gleave, E. Grote, J. Zierski
161 figures. X, 285 pages. 1975. ISBN 3-540-07073-7
Distribution rights for Japan: Maruzen Co. Ltd., Tokyo

Schriftenreihe Neurologie — Neurology Series

Herausgeber: H. J. Bauer, H. Gänshirt, P. Vogel

Vol. 9. M. Wiesendanger: **Pathophysiology of Muscle Tone**
4 figures, VI, 46 pages. 1972. ISBN 3-540-05761-7

Vol. 16. R. Heene: **Experimental Myopathies and Muscular Dystrophy.** Studies in the Formal Pathogenesis of the Myopathy of 2,4-Dichlorophenoxyacetate.
17 figures, VI, 97 pages. 1975. ISBN 3-540-07376-0

Vol. 17. T. Tsuboi, W. Christian: **Epilepsy**
A Clinical, Electroencephalographic, and Statistical Study of 466 Patients.
11 figures, 45 tables, VII, 171 pages. 1976. ISBN 3-540-07735-9

Springer-Verlag
Berlin
Heidelberg
New York

GPSR Compliance
The European Union's (EU) General Product Safety Regulation (GPSR) is a set of rules that requires consumer products to be safe and our obligations to ensure this.

If you have any concerns about our products, you can contact us on

ProductSafety@springernature.com

In case Publisher is established outside the EU, the EU authorized representative is:

Springer Nature Customer Service Center GmbH
Europaplatz 3
69115 Heidelberg, Germany

www.ingramcontent.com/pod-product-compliance
Lightning Source LLC
Chambersburg PA
CBHW080536250926
51846CB00016B/1213
* 9 7 8 3 6 4 2 6 6 5 3 6 3 *